Schizophrenia

Spirits of Schizophrenia and Agoraphobia

(A Simple Guide to Understanding and Managing Schizophrenia)

Royal Cronin

Published By **Region Loviusher**

Royal Cronin

Schizophrenia: Spirits of Schizophrenia and Agoraphobia (A Simple Guide to Understanding and Managing Schizophrenia)

ISBN   978-1-998927-94-4

Legal & Disclaimer

Table Of Contents

Chapter 1: Psychotic Schizophrenia Ailment

Schizophrenia Abnormalities in one or extra of the subsequent 5 domains define them: horrific signs and symptoms and signs, which incorporates delusions, hallucinations, disorganized questioning (collectively with speech), grossly disorganized or uncommon motor conduct (which include catatonia).

KEY ELEMENTS THAT CHARACTERIZE THE CRAZY PROBLEMS

Dreams Hallucinations are everyday convictions that aren't amiable to trade considering clashing proof. Themes together with persecutory, referential, somatic, religious, and grandiose can be covered of their content material cloth. The maximum famous form of persecutory delusions is the perception that an man or woman, corporation, or business company will damage, harass, or otherwise harm them. Referential delusions, additionally referred to as the perception that sure moves, remarks, and environmental cues are geared in the direction of oneself, are also common. Grandiose delusions, moreover referred to as the fake notion that every other person is in love with them, and érotomanie delusions, moreover called the belief that one possesses fantastic abilities, wealth, or reputation, are examples of these varieties of delusions. Skeptical fancies encompass the conviction that a big fiasco will occur, and large hallucinations middle round distractions with regards to wellness and organ functionality. Delusions are taken into consideration weird if they're manifestly improbable, incomprehensible to buddies of the identical lifestyle, and do no longer originate from traditional life opinions. An example of an atypical daydream is the conviction that an outdoor electricity has taken out their indoors organs and supplanted them with some different person's organs without leaving any accidents or scars. The perception that one is below police surveillance no matter the shortage of proof is an example of a non-weird fable. Most people find out bizarre delusions that display a loss of manage over one's thoughts or frame; These embody the belief that one's thoughts were "eliminated" from one's thoughts through an out of doors stress (concept withdrawal), that distant places thoughts have entered one's thoughts (idea insertion), or that one's body or moves are being affected or controlled with the aid of an external strain (delusions of control). The diploma of conviction with which a notion is held regardless of smooth or lower priced contradictory evidence regarding its veracity is one problem that contributes to the hassle in distinguishing a fable from a strongly held idea.

Mind flights Pipedreams are discernment like encounters that occur with out an outer improvement. They are superb and smooth, have the total stress and effect of everyday perceptions, and they may be now not controlled by means of the person. Auditory hallucinations are the most common type of hallucination in schizophrenia and outstanding problems associated with it, but they're able to arise in any sensory mode. Most of the time, auditory hallucinations are professional as voices which is probably perceived as remarkable from the character's own mind, whether or not or now not they may be acquainted or unexpected. The sensorium should be gift for the hallucinations to arise; individuals who take place while one is sleeping (hypnagogic) or waking up (hypnopompic) are taken into consideration to be ordinary. In a few cultural contexts, hallucinations may be a regular part of religious revel in.

Disorganized Thinking (Speech) Disorganized questioning—also known as formal concept illness—is frequently deduced from a person's speech. The individual can also change starting with one issue then onto the subsequent derailment or unfastened affiliations). Questions can be replied in a way that is every tangentially related or completely unrelated (obliqueness). Rarely, speech may be so disordered as to be almost unintelligible, harking back to receptive aphasia in its linguistic illness (incoherence or "word salad"). The symptom have to be excessive enough to significantly keep away from effective conversation because mildly disorganized speech is common and nonspecific. If the man or woman making the diagnosis comes from a unique linguistic historic beyond than the individual being tested, it is able to be hard to evaluate the severity of the impairment. During the prodromal and residual ranges of schizophrenia, disorganized thinking and speech can occur at levels which might be a whole lot less severe.

Horribly Confused or Abnormal Conduct (which includes highbrow marvel) rather disarranged or everyday engine behavior may display itself in diverse strategies, going from sincere "senselessness" to capricious tumult. Any motive-directed behavior might also additionally have troubles that make it difficult to carry out each day sports. A marked decrease in reactivity to the surroundings is catatonic behavior. This reaches from safety from pointers negativism); to keeping an atypical, inflexible, or irrelevant posture; to mutism and stupor, a whole loss of motor and verbal responses). Catatonic exhilaration) also can embody irrational and excessive motor interest and now not the usage of a apparent cause. The mutism, repeated stereotyped moves, staring, grimacing, and speech echoing are extra traits. Catatonia symptoms and signs and signs and symptoms are nonspecific and may stand up in other highbrow problems (alongside aspect bipolar or depressive issues with catatonia) and clinical conditions, no matter the fact that catatonia has traditionally been associated with schizophrenia.

Negative Symptoms even though they will be less common in distinctive psychotic issues, terrible symptoms and signs and symptoms make up a massive part of the morbidity associated with schizophrenia. Schizophrenia is characterised with the beneficial resource of especially exquisite horrible symptoms and signs: faded functionality for emotional expression and idea. The face, eye contact, intonation of speech (prosody), and actions of the hand, head, and face that normally provide an emotional emphasis to speech are all examples of dwindled emotional expression. There is a decline in self-triggered, sensible sports activities which is probably self-initiated. The man or woman would possibly likely take a seat for a long term and show little hobby in going for walks or having fun with buddies. Alogia, anhedonia, and asociality are additional terrible signs and signs. Alogia can be seen in reduced speech output. Anhedonia is the disability to enjoy delight from high fantastic stimuli or a decline inside the capacity to remember pride that has been professional previously. Avolition and asociality may be linked to an obvious lack of hobby in social interactions, but asociality also can advocate a loss of possibilities for social interactions.

This chapter is organized in a psychopathological gradient. Conditions that do not meet all the standards for a psychotic illness or which might be constrained to a unmarried psychopathology need to be taken into consideration first with the aid of clinicians. Then they must consider conditions with constrained time. Lastly, as a way to make a diagnosis of schizophrenia spectrum disorder, each other condition that could purpose psychosis have to be ruled out. Although its full description can be positioned inside the financial disaster titled "Personality Disorders," schizotypal character illness is cited on this bankruptcy due to the fact it's miles protected in the schizophrenia spectrum. A large pattern of social and interpersonal deficits, which encompass a diminished capability for close to relationships, is captured through way of the evaluation of schizotypal character sickness. Distortions of concept or notion; and eccentricities in conduct, which usually start in early adulthood however may also furthermore initially appear in adolescence and adolescence in a few times. A psychotic infection can't be identified based totally on ideals, thoughts, or perceptions which can be everyday. Two activities are characterised via way of the usage of irregularities constrained to at least one area of psychosis: catatonia or delusions Delusional ailment is characterised via using having delusions for as a minimum one month with out unique psychotic signs. Catatonia is cited in addition on this dialogue and later inside the financial break. A brief psychotic disorder lasts for more than one day and disappears after one month. The signs and signs of schizophrenia-like schizophreniform illness are much like the ones of schizophrenia, with the exception of the infection's brief length (plenty less than six months) and the absence of a requirement for a decline in functioning. At least one month of lively-phase symptoms and symptoms are required for schizophrenia to very last for as a minimum six months. A temper episode and the lively-phase symptoms and symptoms of schizophrenia rise up concurrently in schizoaffective illness, and the mood episode have emerge as preceded or found via as a minimum weeks of delusions or hallucinations without prominent mood signs and signs. Another condition might also furthermore motive psychotic issues. Psychotic symptoms and symptoms in substance/medication-caused psychotic sickness are idea to be a physiological cease result of publicity to a drug of abuse, remedy, or pollutants and go away even as the agent is eliminated. Psychotic signs and symptoms are considered to be a right away physiological impact of another scientific state of affairs in psychotic sickness due to every distinct situation. Neurodevelopmental, psychotic, bipolar, depressive, and one-of-a-type highbrow issues all have the ability to cause catatonia. Catatonia related to a few distinctive intellectual illness (catatonia specifier), catatonic disorder due to each specific scientific situation, and unspecified catatonia are all diagnoses that are stated in this bankruptcy. The diagnostic requirements for each of these 3 situations are stated collectively. For the motive of classifying psychotic suggests that do not meet the necessities for any of the unique psychotic troubles or psychotic symptomatology about which there is inadequate or contradictory information, different certain and unspecified

11

schizophrenia spectrum and other psychotic troubles are blanketed.

Evaluation of Psychosis Symptoms and Related Clinical Phenomena with the aid of the use of Clinicians the severity of symptoms of psychotic issues can expect essential elements of the infection, which encompass the diploma of cognitive or neurobiological deficits, which might be severa. "Assessment Measures," a complete framework for severity evaluation is covered to increase the sector. This framework can be useful for remedy planning, prognostic desire-making, and research on pathophysiological mechanisms. Dimensional tests of the number one signs and symptoms and symptoms of psychosis, collectively with hallucinations, delusions, disorganized speech (other than substance/scientific-brought on psychotic contamination and psychotic illness due to each other medical situation), everyday psychomotor conduct, and bad signs and symptoms and signs and symptoms, also are covered in Section III, this is titled "Assessment Measures." Dimensional assessments of depression and mania are also blanketed. In psychosis, the severity of temper symptoms and signs and symptoms has prognostic fee and directs remedy. The loss of a first-rate nosological class for schizoaffective illness is becoming more and more obvious. Subsequently, layered fee determinations of distress and madness for all loopy issues organized clinicians to temperament pathology and the need to cope with wherein turning into. A lot of people with psychotic problems have deficits in plenty of cognitive domain names that can are waiting for how useful they will be. Although brief checks that don't contain a proper neuropsychological evaluation can offer beneficial facts that can be enough for diagnostic abilties, scientific neuropsychological assessment can assist in guiding analysis and treatment. Formal neuropsychological trying out, even as led,

13

need to be managed and scored by using way of the use of artwork stress prepared within the usage of trying out devices. The clinician want to choose based truely on the most accurate statistics to be had inside the absence of a proper neuropsychological assessment. It may be vital to behavior extra studies on those checks to decide their clinical application; The necessities and textual content for the schizotypal persona illness may be found inside the "Personality Disorders" bankruptcy. This sickness is indexed on this chapter and mentioned in detail in the DSM-5 bankruptcy "Personality Disorders" due to the fact it's far included inside the schizophrenia spectrum of issues and is referred to as schizotypal disorder on this section of ICD-9 and ICD-10. Diagnostic

CRITERIA FOR DELUSIONAL DISORDERS

1. The presence of 1 or extra delusions lasting at the least one month.

2 Schizophrenia has by no means fulfilled criterion A. Note: If hallucinations are gift, they may be minor and related to the delusional subject (as an example, delusions of infestation are associated with the sensation of being infested with insects).

3. Other than the effect of the fantasy or fable(s) or its repercussions, functioning isn't always notably impaired, and behavior is not absolutely uncommon or bizarre.

four. In assessment to the duration of the delusional periods, any episodes of manic or maximum crucial depressive disorder that have happened had been brief.

five. The disturbance isn't always better defined with the resource of the use of some other intellectual disorder, which encompass frame dysmorphic sickness or obsessive-compulsive illness, and it isn't always because of the physiological effects of a substance or some other scientific situation.

Indicate whether or not or now not or no longer: Type of Erotomanie: When the fable's applicable theme is that each unique person is in love with the character, this subtype applies. Type grandiose: When the important subject matter of the myth is the conviction that one possesses massive information, notion, or abilities that isn't always identified, this subtype applies. Type of jerk: When someone's essential fable is that their partner or lover is cheating on them, they fall into this subtype. Type of persecutor: When the man or woman's notion that she or he is being conspired closer to, cheated, spied on, located, poisoned or drugged, maliciously maligned, stressed, or obstructed inside the pursuit of prolonged-term goals is the crucial topic of the myth, this subtype applies. Substantial kind: When the myth's valuable problem includes physical features or sensations, this subtype applies. Types blended: When there can be no unmarried delusional issue be counted that dominates, this subtype applies. Type not particular: Referential delusions with out a remarkable persecutory or grandiose component, as an example, fall into this subtype at the same time as the dominant delusional belief is both not genuinely defined or can not be decided. Indicate if: with outlandish content cloth: A person's notion that a stranger has eliminated their inner organs and modified them with the organs of every other person with out leaving any wounds or scars is an example of a peculiar fantasy this is virtually awesome, unintelligible, and now not derived from everyday lifestyles research. Indicate if: After 3 hundred and sixty five days of the sickness, brilliant the following path specifiers may be used: First episode, right now in extreme episode: First sign of the problem assembly the characterizing indicative factor effect and time requirements. A time whilst the symptom standards are met is known as an acute episode. First episode, it is now partially under control: The time period "partial remission" refers to a time period wherein the sickness's defining developments are handiest in factor met at the same time as an improvement from a previous episode is maintained. First episode, that is now truly lengthy beyond: A time frame following a previous episode on the same time as there are not any disease-unique signs and signs and symptoms is called whole remission. Multiple episodes which might be presently in acute section more than one episodes which is probably in part remission multiple episodes which may be genuinely remission subthreshold symptom intervals are relatively short in assessment to the infection's widespread course, but signs and symptoms that meet the sickness's diagnostic criteria persist at a few diploma in the majority of its path. Undetermined Describe the present day severity: A quantitative evaluation of the primary symptoms of psychosis—delusions, hallucinations, disorganized speech, peculiar psychomotor behavior, and terrible symptoms and signs—is used to determine severity. On a five-thing scale that degrees from zero (now not gift) to four (gift and excessive), each of those symptoms and symptoms and symptoms may be rated regular with its modern-day severity (maximum intense inside the last seven days). In the financial disaster titled "Assessment Measures," you could find out Clinician-Rated Dimensions of Psychosis Symptom Severity.) Note: It is viable to make a evaluation of delusional sickness with out the usage of this severity specifier. Subtypes In the érotomanie type, the notion that each different man or woman is in love with the man or woman is the important situation be counted wide variety of the myth. This conviction is generally held about someone of higher fame, like a well-known man or woman or a superior at work, however it may also be approximately a person simply unknown. Common is the attempt to get in contact with the delusional item. In the grandiose kind, the delusion's primary issue remember is the conviction that the character has good sized perception, expertise, or discovery. In less commonplace times, the individual may additionally moreover trust they will be a well-known character or have a completely specific courting with a famous individual (in which case the real man or woman can be seen as an impostor). There can be spiritual underpinnings to grandiose delusions. In inexperienced with envy type, the focal issue rely of the dream is that of an untrustworthy partner. This perception is derived erroneously and is supported through insignificant portions of "evidence" (which encompass garb in disarray). Typically, the person who has the myth confronts their accomplice or lover and tries to intrude in the imagined infidelity. The character's belief that they'll be being conspired against, cheated, spied on, located, poisoned, maliciously maligned, careworn, or obstructed inside the pursuit of extended-time period desires is the important concern of the persecutory sort of fable. A delusional tool may additionally moreover cognizance on minor offenses and exaggerate them. The affected person also can try to get what they need via way of way of taking jail or legislative movement again and again. People who've persecutory delusions often sense resentment and rage, and they'll even use violence towards those they remember are causing them harm. The body's capabilities or sensations are the treasured project recall of somatic delusion. There are many specific sorts of somatic delusions. The most mounted concept is that the individual offers off an unpleasant perfume; that there are insects infesting the pores and skin or on it; that an inner parasite exists; that a few components of the body are not right or appearance awful; or that a few body factors are not operating right? Diagnostic Characteristics the presence of 1 or greater delusions that last for at the least a month is the maximum critical function of delusional sickness

(Criterion A). If someone has ever presented with symptoms and symptoms and signs and symptoms that meet Criteria A for schizophrenia (Criterion B), they may be not given a evaluation of delusional ailment. In addition to having a direct effect from the delusions, the impairments in psychosocial functioning can be extra confined than in unique psychotic problems like schizophrenia, and the behavior is not outright first-rate or weird (Criterion C). According to Criteria D, if temper episodes stand up concurrently with delusions, their basic period is shorter than that of the delusional periods. The delusions aren't higher defined through the use of a few other intellectual disorder, at the side of frame dysmorphic disease or obsessive-compulsive ailment (Criterion E), nor are they due to the physiological consequences of a substance like cocaine or each different scientific situation like Alzheimer's disorder.

For making crucial variations among the severa schizophrenia spectrum problems and super psychotic troubles, the evaluation of cognition, despair, and mania symptom domain names is vital in addition to the five symptom area areas recognized within the diagnostic standards.

Delusional beliefs in delusional sickness can cause social, marital, or artwork troubles. Associated Features Supporting Diagnosis in spite of the reality that they'll have "genuine insight" however no true perception, human beings with delusional ailment may be able to factually describe that others view their ideals as irrational. Many human beings revel in temper swings like irritability or dysphoria because of their delusional ideals. Persecutory, jealous, and érotomanie kinds can purpose anger and violent behavior. The individual can also act in a adverse (as an example, via the use of using writing loads of letters of protest to the authorities).

Legal troubles can rise up, especially in jealousy and érotomania.

Prevalence the maximum common subtype of delusional disorder, persecutory, has an entire lifestyles incidence of approximately zero.2%. Although there are not any large gender variations within the popular frequency of delusional illness, the jealous form of delusional disorder might be greater commonplace in individual guys than in females.

Development and Course Global function generally performs higher than in schizophrenia on commonplace. Despite the fact that the assessment is typically strong, some people bypass directly to increase schizophrenia. Schizophrenia and schizotypal character disorder percent a fantastic familial reference to delusional disorder. The condition can have an effect on people of every age, but it can be greater common in older humans.

Chapter 2: Obsessive-Compulsive Disorder Differential Diagnosis

Obsessive-compulsive illness and its comorbid situations. Instead of a evaluation of delusional ailment, the analysis of obsessive-compulsive illness with absent belief/delusional beliefs specifier need to get hold of to a person who's genuinely glad that their obsessive-compulsive disorder ideals are right. Similarly, a evaluation of body dysmorphic sickness with absent insight/delusional ideals specifier ought to take shipping of in region of a analysis of delusional disease if a person with body dysmorphic disease is truely happy that their frame dysmorphic sickness beliefs are real. Delirium, fundamental neurocognitive disease, psychotic disorder introduced on via any other medical situation, and psychotic illness introduced on through materials or medicinal tablets. People with those issues may additionally moreover deliver component outcomes that endorse fanciful confusion. In the context of fundamental neurocognitive ailment, for instance, simple persecutory delusions might be classified as essential neurocognitive disorder with behavioral disturbance. Cross-sectional, a substance- or medication-triggered psychotic sickness might also moreover share symptoms with delusional disease, but it could be great through the chronological relationship the numerous onset and remission of delusions. Schizophreniform disease and schizophrenia. The absence of the opportunity defining symptoms and signs and symptoms of the energetic segment of schizophrenia distinguishes delusional ailment from schizophrenia and schizophreniform illness. Schizoaffective illness, bipolar contamination, and depression. The severity of the temper signs and signs and symptoms and the temporal relationship a number of the mood disturbance and the delusions can assist distinguish these troubles from delusional illness. Depressive or bipolar illness with psychotic capabilities is the diagnosis if delusions handiest stand up at some point of temper swings. Delusional infection can be layered on pinnacle of mood symptoms and signs and symptoms and signs that meet the whole definition of a temper episode. Only if the entire duration of all temper episodes is shorter than the whole length of the delusional disturbance can a analysis of delusional disease be made. Other precise or unspecified schizophrenia spectrum and exclusive psychotic sickness, along aspect different precise depressive sickness, unspecified depressive disorder, other unique bipolar and related sickness, or unspecified bipolar and associated illness, is suitable if this is not the case.

SHORT PSYCHOTIC DISORDER DIAGNOSTIC CRITERIA 298.Eight (F23)

The presence of 1 or greater of the symptoms listed under. It should be as a minimum one of the following:

1. Delusions.

2. Hallucinations.

three. Speech disorder (which incorporates not unusual detours or incoherence)

four. Utterly chaotic or disorganized conduct.

Note: If a symptom is a culturally right response, you want to no longer encompass it.

An episode of the disturbance lasts for at least eventually but lots much less than a month, with a whole cross lower again to pre-morbid functioning eventually taking place.

The unsettling have an effect on isn't better made experience of through massive burdensome or bipolar turmoil with crazy factors or some other insane problem like schizophrenia or highbrow wonder, and isn't because of the physiological impacts of a substance (e.G., a medicine of misuse, a drug) or a few specific illness.

Indicate if: With super stressors (brief-term reactive psychosis): If signs and signs and signs and symptoms rise up because of occasions that, each on their private or in mixture, could be extraordinarily annoying for almost all and sundry in the identical situation within the character's manner of existence. Stressors in absence of marriage: If signs and signs and signs do no longer upward thrust up in reaction to sports that, every in my view or together, is probably extremely demanding for almost all of us inside the person's lifestyle who well-knownshows themselves in similar occasions, Beginning postpartum: if it begins in the course of being pregnant or inside four weeks of giving begin. Indicate if: With catatonia (see the pp. Standards for catatonia with some one of a kind intellectual sickness). To suggest the presence of the comorbid catatonia, use extra code 293.89 (F06.1) catatonia related to short psychotic disorder.

Please specify the severity within the meantime: A quantitative assessment of the number one symptoms and symptoms of psychosis—delusions, hallucinations, disorganized speech, regular psychomotor conduct, and horrible signs and symptoms— is used to determine severity. On a 5-element scale that ranges from 0 (now not gift) to 4 (present and excessive), every of those signs and symptoms can be rated constant with its present day severity (most excessive within the very last seven days). In the chapter titled "Assessment Measures," you may discover Clinician-Rated Dimensions of Psychosis Symptom Severity.) Note: It is possible to make a analysis of brief psychotic illness without the use of this severity specifier.

Diagnostic Characteristics A disturbance characterised via the sudden onset of at least one of the following effective psychotic signs and symptoms is the primary function of brief psychotic illness. Disorganized speech (consisting of not unusual derailment or incoherence) or certainly weird psychomotor behavior, together with catatonia (Criterion A). Change from a nonpsychotic nation to a absolutely psychotic kingdom internal two weeks, commonly without a prodrome, is known as sudden onset. A disturbance episode lasts for at least subsequently but now not more than one month, and the character in the end returns surely to their pre-morbid kingdom of functioning (Criteria B). The disturbance is not as a consequence of the physiological consequences of a substance (at the aspect of a hallucinogen) or every different medical state of affairs (which incorporates a subdural hematoma) and can't be better described by way of the use of a depressive illness, bipolar disease with psychotic abilities, schizoaffective ailment, or schizophrenia (Criterion C). For making vital differences maximum of the severa schizophrenia spectrum troubles and other psychotic issues, the assessment of cognition, depression, and mania symptom domains is essential in addition to the 5 symptom area areas diagnosed in the diagnostic necessities.

Related Highlights Supporting Analysis People with brief maniacal problem generally enjoy inner disturbance or overpowering disarray. They may also trade from one intense have an effect directly to some other speedy. Even although the disturbance is brief, the quantity of impairment can be excessive, and supervision can be required to ensure that the character is blanketed from the results of terrible judgment, cognitive impairment, or appearing on delusions similarly to that the nutritional and hygienic goals are met. During the extreme episode, there appears to be an expanded hazard of suicidal behavior.

Prevalence within the United States, brief psychotic illness may additionally moreover cause first-onset psychosis in nine% of humans. Developing nations outnumber advanced worldwide places with regards to the prevalence of psychotic disturbances that meet Criteria A and C, however not Criteria B, for quick psychotic ailment (i.E., active signs and symptoms and signs and symptoms ultimate among one and six months as opposed to remission indoors one month). Females have a twofold better occurrence of short psychotic illness than guys do.

The onset of development and route brief psychotic illness can occur at any age, with the median age of onset being in the mid-30s. It can arise in adolescence or early maturity. A short psychotic sickness assessment necessitates a whole remission of all signs and symptoms and an eventual whole go back to pre-morbid functioning inner one month of the disturbance's onset.

The period of psychotic signs and symptoms and signs in a few human beings can be quite quick (some days, for example).

CHARACTERISTICS OF RISIC AND PROGNOSTIC FACTORS

Traits and individual issues which is probably already gift (as an instance, schizotypal personality illness; marginal behavioral circumstance; or on the other hand trends inside the psychoticism area, like perceptual dysregulation, and the terrible affectivity area, like dubiousness) might also incline the man or woman towards the improvement of the hassle.

Culture-Related Diagnostic issues it is important to differentiate between culturally normal response patterns and signs of brief psychotic illness. For example, in some strict abilties, an person could in all likelihood record being attentive to voices, however the ones don't via and large go through and are not seen as ordinary via maximum humans from the singular's network vicinity. When figuring out whether or not or not or no longer ideals are delusional, cultural and religious records ought to moreover be taken into consideration.

Functional Consequences of Brief Psycliotic Disorder Despite the immoderate price of relapse, most patients collect superb results in phrases of symptomatology and social functioning.

DIFFERENTIAL PSYCHOTIC DIAGNOSIS

Psychotic signs and symptoms can be short manifestations of numerous clinical conditions. When there's evidence from the affected character's statistics, physical examination, or laboratory exams that the delusions or hallucinations are the direct physiological impact of a selected medical state of affairs (which include Cushing's syndrome or a mind tumor), psychotic ailment due to each extraordinary scientific circumstance or delirium is recognized (see "Tsychotic Disorder Due to Another Medical Condition" later on this financial ruin). Disorders because of tablets. Substance/medicine-precipitated psychotic contamination, substance-induced delirium, and substance intoxication are outstanding from brief psychotic illness in that a substance (which include an abuse drug, remedy, or publicity to a toxins) is taken into consideration to be etiologically related to the psychotic signs (see "Substance/Medication-Induced Psychotic Disorder" later in this financial disaster). A careful records of substance use, paying specific attention to the temporal relationships among substance intake and onset of signs and the character of the substance being used, may also be useful in making this self-control. Laboratory checks like a urine drug show show or a blood alcohol degree will also be useful. Bipolar and depressive issues. If the psychotic signs and symptoms are better described by way of the use of a temper episode (i.E., they wonderful occur sooner or later of a full critical depressive, manic, or combined episode), a analysis of brief psychotic ailment can't be made. Other intellectual illnesses. Depending on the alternative symptoms gift, the diagnosis is each schizophreniform illness, delusional sickness, despair with psychotic capabilities, bipolar disorder with psychotic capabilities, or each other precise or unspecified schizophrenia spectrum and other psychotic illness if the psychotic symptoms and signs and symptoms and symptoms persist for as a minimum one month. When the psychotic signs and symptoms and symptoms have subsided in advance than one month in response to a fulfillment medicinal drug treatment, it's miles difficult to distinguish amongst brief psychotic sickness and schizophreniform disorder. The possibility that any recurrent psychotic episodes are due to a recurrent disorder (which include bipolar illness or recurrent acute exacerbations of schizophrenia) need to be cautiously considered. Disorders of malingering and factuality. It is feasible for a quick psychotic sickness to seem as an episode of factitious sickness with regularly intellectual signs and symptoms and symptoms and signs; however, there is evidence that the signs and signs had been deliberately produced in such instances. There is usually proof that the contamination is being feigned for an comprehensible purpose when malingering consists of signs and signs that look like psychotic. Behavioral situations. Psychosocial stressors can reason brief episodes of psychotic signs and symptoms and signs in a few human beings with character problems. Since those symptoms and signs and symptoms are typically short, they do not necessitate a separate evaluation. A 2nd diagnosis of quick psychotic sickness can be essential if psychotic signs and signs closing for at least in the destiny.

Diagnostic Characteristics The signs and symptoms and symptoms and signs of schizophreniform infection (Criterion A) are same to the ones of schizophrenia. The duration of schizophrenia is what devices it other than specific highbrow fitness conditions: the contamination lasts for at the least one month but not greater than six months regular, along with the prodromal, energetic, and residual stages (Criterion B). Schizophreniform infection has a period requirement this is someplace in among that of schizophrenia, which lasts at least six months, and quick psychotic illness, which lasts for added than a day and goes away in a month. There are requirements for creating a schizophreniform illness evaluation. 1) whilst an illness episode lasts among one and 6 months and the character has recovered; 2) on the identical time as someone is symptomatic for much less than the six months required for a schizophrenia prognosis but has not recovered. Because it's far unsure whether or not the person will get over the disturbance within six months, the diagnosis want to be "schizophreniform disorder (provisional)" on this example. The evaluation have to be modified to schizophrenia if the disturbance keeps for longer than six months.

The absence of a criterion requiring impairment in social and occupational functioning is a few other distinguishing feature of schizophreniform disease. Although such impairments can be gift, they're not important for a schizophreniform ailment diagnosis. For making essential variations the diverse various schizophrenia spectrum problems and different psychotic troubles, the evaluation of cognition, despair, and mania symptom domain names is vital further to the 5 symptom place areas diagnosed inside the diagnostic requirements.

The absence of psychometric or laboratory assessments for schizophreniform sickness is much like that of schizophrenia and allows the analysis. Neuroimaging, neurophysiological, and neurological research have located abnormalities in some of thoughts regions, but none are diagnostic.

Prevalence even though there's said variation via race/ethnicity, throughout international locations, and through manner of geographic foundation for immigrants and children of immigrants, the lifetime occurrence of schizophrenia seems to be between 0.Three% and zero.7%. The gender ratio varies among populations and samples: as an example, an accentuation on regrettable factor effects and longer length of turmoil (associated with masses much less lucky end end result) shows higher frequency expenses for guys, although definitions thinking about the incorporation of additional temperament issue effects and brief introductions (associated with improved give up result) show similar dangers for the two genders.

Development and Course Schizophrenia's psychotic symptoms and symptoms usually start in the past due teenagers or early 30s; onset in advance than young adults is uncommon. For adult grownup males, the height age at which the primary psychotic episode starts offevolved offevolved is inside the early to mid-20s, at the equal time as for ladies, it's far in the past due 20s. Although the majority of humans experience a gradual and sluggish onset of an entire lot of clinically big symptoms and signs and signs and signs and symptoms, the onset may be unexpected or subtle. Half of those human beings say they've signs and symptoms and symptoms of melancholy. In the past, it has been concept that a worse analysis is related to an earlier age at onset. However, guys are likely to have a worse premorbid adjustment, decrease instructional success, extra fantastic bad signs and symptoms, and cognitive impairment, in addition to a worse outcome common, due to the impact of age at onset.

Disabled notion is regular, and changes in comprehension are available during improvement and pass in advance than the improvement of psychosis, performing as consistent intellectual debilitations within the path of adulthood. Mental impedances might possibly persevere whilst super detail results are going away and upload to the disability of the contamination. Course and very last effects predictors are in large part unidentified, and they may not be reliably anticipated. About 20% of people with schizophrenia appear to revel in the remedy, and a small percentage are stated to certainly recover. However, the majority of human beings with schizophrenia though require both formal or casual enables for each day dwelling, and a few be afflicted by modern deterioration on the same time as others experience persistent infection with exacerbations and remissions of lively signs. Psychotic signs and symptoms and signs and signs and symptoms generally will be predisposed to go away through the years, likely collectively with the ordinary decline in dopamine hobby that includes age. Negative signs and symptoms and signs and signs commonly ultimate longer and are greater closely associated with assessment than extremely good signs. Additionally, it's viable that the contamination's cognitive impairments will no longer depart. Although it is more tough to diagnose schizophrenia in adolescence, the precept symptoms and signs continue to be the equal. Visual hallucinations are more common in kids than in adults, and they need to be splendid from regular delusion play. Delusions and hallucinations may be lots less complex in youngsters than in adults. Disorganized behavior and speech are commonplace manifestations of many adolescence-onset troubles, together with hobby-deficit/hyperactivity ailment (ADHD). Without considering the more significant issues of formative years, it's far beside the factor to attribute these symptoms and symptoms and symptoms to schizophrenia.

With a gradual onset and splendid terrible signs, times with adolescents onset generally resemble adult cases with terrible results. Nonspecific emotional-behavioral disturbances and psychopathology, intellectual and language modifications, and diffused motor delays are more not unusual in children who later receive a schizophrenia analysis. Females, who may moreover furthermore have married, make up the majority of instances with overdue-onset (onset after age forty). The direction frequently is composed extensively talking of psychotic signs and symptoms at the same time as maintaining have an effect on and social functioning. Although the ones past due-onset instances can nonetheless meet the requirements for schizophrenia analysis, it isn't but clean whether or no longer or now not they will be the same as schizophrenia identified earlier than midlife (as an instance, earlier than age 55).

Chapter 3: Environmental Risk And Prognostic Factors

The onset of schizophrenia has been linked to the time of yr of delivery, with the deficit shape taking vicinity in summer time in a few regions and late winter/early spring in others. Children from urban regions and a few minority ethnic agencies are more likely to develop schizophrenia and associated problems. Biological and genetic factors. Despite the truth that almost all of people who have been diagnosed with schizophrenia do now not have a statistics of psychosis in their households, genetic elements play a big function in identifying risk for schizophrenia. A sort of danger alleles, both common and uncommon, confer criminal obligation, with each allele most effective contributing a small a part of the general populace variance. Bipolar disease, melancholy, and autism spectrum disorder are all related to the danger alleles which have been diagnosed so far. Pregnancy and birth entanglements with hypoxia and further first rate fatherly age are associated with a higher gamble of schizophrenia for the developing embryo. Stress, contamination, malnutrition, maternal diabetes, and a whole lot of other prenatal and perinatal adversities have additionally been linked to schizophrenia. However, schizophrenia does now not occur within the enormous majority of offspring with the ones risk elements.

Cultural and socioeconomic factors need to be taken into consideration while diagnosing a affected character, specifically if the patient and the clinical clinical physician do not come from the identical cultural and socioeconomic ancient beyond. In one culture, beliefs that seem like illogical, like witchcraft, can be appreciably held in every other. Visual or auditory hallucinations with non secular content cloth material, along with listening to God's voice, are common spiritual reviews in a few cultures. Language variations in narrative styles amongst cultures can also make it hard to assess disorganized speech. Sensitivity to cultural variations in emotional expression, eye touch, and body language is important for affect assessment. Care have to be taken to avoid alogia due to linguistic barriers if the evaluation is finished in a language other than the person's nearby tongue. In some cultures, misery can appear as hallucinations or pseudo-hallucinations in addition to overvalued mind that would look like real psychosis from a scientific perspective but are commonplace most of the affected individual's subgroup.

Gender-Related Diagnostic Problems There are some distinguishing developments most of the clinical manifestations of schizophrenia in women and men. Females will be predisposed to have a barely lower standard occurrence of schizophrenia, particularly in treated times. Females experience a later age of onset and a 2d midlife top, as formerly said (for added records on this illness, see the section titled "Development and Course"). Females have more have an effect on-laden symptoms and signs and symptoms and signs, more psychotic symptoms, and a greater propensity for psychotic signs and symptoms and signs to get worse over the years.

Negative symptoms that are much less common and disorganization are extra variations in signs and symptoms. Last however now not least, women are more likely to maintain their social functioning. There are, nevertheless, non-stop unique cases for those common provisos.

Suicide Risic Between 5% and 6% of humans with schizophrenia dedicate suicide, 20% make at least one suicide strive, and masses of greater have sizable suicidal thoughts. Sometimes, command hallucinations to harm oneself or others purpose suicidal behavior. Both males and females face a high risk of suicide in the direction of their entire lives, despite the fact that greater younger guys who have a facts of substance abuse issues may be specially inclined. Having depressive signs and symptoms or feelings of hopelessness, being unemployed, and experiencing a psychotic episode or health facility discharge are extra danger elements.

The purposeful consequences of schizophrenia include giant social and expert dysfunction. Even whilst cognitive capabilities are sufficient for the duties at hand, avolition or other disease manifestations regularly impair educational development and employment. The majority of humans, particularly men, do now not marry and feature few social connections outside of their own family, and their employment levels are lower than those in their mother and father.

Major depressive or bipolar illness with psychotic or catatonic signs and symptoms is a differential prognosis. The temporal courting most of the mood disturbance and the psychosis, further to the severity of the depressive or manic signs and signs, decide the difference among schizophrenia and vital depressive or bipolar disease with psychotic capabilities or catatonia. In the occasion that daydreams or pipedreams seem completely at some stage in a widespread burdensome or hyper episode, the power of will is burdensome or bipolar confusion with loopy factors. Disorder of schizophrenia. A crucial depressive or manic episode have to arise concurrently with lively-segment signs on the manner to be identified with schizoaffective ailment, and temper signs and symptoms and signs and symptoms ought to be gift for nearly all of the energetic periods. Short-time period psychotic ailment and schizophrenia. According to Criterion C, these troubles final lots less time than schizophrenia, which calls for 6 months of signs. The disturbance in schizophreniform ailment lasts a great deal much much less than six months, on the identical time as in quick psychotic sickness, symptoms final as a minimum sooner or later however a good deal much less than one month. Disorder of the delusions Other signs and symptoms and signs of schizophrenia, which incorporates delusions, incredible auditory or seen hallucinations, disorganized speech, grossly disorganized or catatonic conduct, and negative signs, are absent in delusional sickness, which distinguishes it from schizophrenia. Disorder of the schizotypal person subthreshold signs and signs and symptoms which may be associated with chronic persona tendencies can set schizophrenia apart from schizotypal man or woman disease. Body dysmorphic disease and obsessive-compulsive sickness. Obsessive-compulsive sickness and body dysmorphic sickness sufferers also can moreover present with or without restricted notion, and their problems might also additionally reap delusional proportions. However, the distinguished obsessions, compulsions, preoccupations with look or frame fragrance, hoarding, and body-targeted repetitive behaviors that the ones problems display off set them other than schizophrenia. Disorder of post-worrying stress. Hypervigilance can achieve paranoid proportions in posttraumatic stress disease, and flashbacks that have the extremely good of hallucinations are a probable problem. However, that allows you to make a analysis, a traumatic occasion and particular symptoms and signs associated with reliving or responding to the occasion are required. Disorders of communique or the autism spectrum those troubles are high-quality by manner of way in their respective deficits in social interaction, which incorporates restricted and repetitive behaviors as well as different cognitive and verbal exchange deficits. They might also furthermore display off symptoms and signs and symptoms which may be just like those of a psychotic episode. An man or woman with highbrow imbalance range confusion or correspondence hassle want to have side effects that meet entire requirements for schizophrenia, with unmistakable fantasies or goals for a few issue like multi month, to be decided to have schizophrenia as a comorbid situation. Other intellectual ailments which might be linked to a psychotic episode. Only while the psychotic episode lasts for an extended term and isn't always due to the physiological outcomes of a substance or a few distinctive scientific circumstance can the prognosis of schizophrenia be made. People with a ridiculousness or number one or minor neurocognitive trouble might probably supply insane element results, however those might have a brief dating to the begin of intellectual changes consistent with the ones problems. Criterion A symptoms and signs and signs for schizophrenia may be determined in people with substance/medicinal drug-added about psychotic sickness; however, the substance/medicinal drug-delivered about psychotic disorder is usually prominent via the chronological relationship a few of the onset and remission of the psychosis inside the absence of substance use.

Schizophrenia has a excessive fee of comorbidity with substance-associated problems. Over 1/2 of of people with schizophrenia smoke cigarettes on a ordinary foundation and be tormented by the usage of a tobacco use ailment. Schizophrenia is becoming an increasing number of related to anxiety issues. When in assessment to the overall populace, individuals with schizophrenia have better fees of OCD and panic troubles. Paranoid or schizophrenic individual infection can every so often upward thrust up earlier than schizophrenia. Due to the related scientific situations, schizophrenia patients have a shorter life expectancy. Diabetes, metabolic syndrome, cardiovascular and pulmonary sickness, in addition to weight gain, are more normal in schizophrenia sufferers than in the trendy populace. Chronic disorder is more likely to get up if people don't do matters to maintain their fitness in test, like getting screened for cancer or exercising, however there are other factors like drug treatments, lifestyle, smoking, and food plan that could furthermore play a position. Some of schizophrenia's scientific comorbidity can be described by way of the use of a shared vulnerability to psychosis and scientific troubles.

A non-stop period of contamination wherein there can be a high temper episode (essential depressive or manic) concurrent with Criterion A of schizophrenia is a schizophrenic contamination. Note: Criterion A1 of the essential depressive episode want to be gift: Feeling down. B. Delusions or hallucinations lasting or more weeks without a top temper episode (depressive or manic) all through the contamination's lifetime. C. During the bulk of the infection's energetic and residual tiers, signs and symptoms and symptoms that meet the requirements for a outstanding temper episode are present. D. The disturbance is unrelated to the effects of a substance (which incorporates a treatment or substance of abuse) or a clinical scenario.

Indicate whether or not or no longer: 295.70 (F25.Zero) Type of bipolar: If the presentation includes a manic episode, this subtype applies. Significant burdensome episodes might also moreover likewise appear. 295.70 (F25.1) Type of melancholy: If the presentation great consists of number one depressive episodes, this subtype applies. Indicate if: With catatonia (see the pp. Standards for catatonia with each different intellectual sickness). For a definition, see 119-120). Note for code: To endorse the presence of the comorbid catatonia, use additional code 293.89 (F06.1) catatonia associated with schizoaffective ailment.

Indicate if: The following path specifiers need to most effective be used after the illness has been gift for at least 3 hundred and sixty five days and if they do no longer battle with the diagnostic direction necessities. Acute episode presently in its first section: first signal or symptom of the disorder that meets the time and defining diagnostic symptom necessities. A time while the symptom standards are met is referred to as an acute episode. First episode, that is now partly underneath control: The term "partial remission" refers to a time body wherein the sickness's defining developments are top notch partly met whilst an development from a preceding episode is maintained. First episode, it's now truely long gone: A time period following a previous episode on the same time as there aren't any illness-specific signs is called whole remission. Several episodes, currently in acute: After as a minimum episodes (i.E., a first episode, a remission, and at the least one relapse), more than one episodes can be determined. Several episodes which might be presently in partial remission Several episodes which might be currently in full remission Subthreshold symptom durations are quite brief in evaluation to the infection's commonplace course, however signs and symptoms and symptoms and signs and symptoms that meet the sickness's diagnostic requirements persist throughout the bulk of its direction. Undetermined Describe the modern-day severity: A quantitative assessment of the number one signs and signs and signs and symptoms of psychosis—delusions, hallucinations, disorganized speech, remarkable psychomotor behavior, and poor symptoms and signs and symptoms and signs—is used to determine severity. On a 5-factor scale that tiers from zero (not gift) to 4 (gift and immoderate), each of those signs can be rated constant with its current severity (most excessive in the final seven days). In the monetary catastrophe titled

"Assessment Measures," you can discover Clinician-Rated Dimensions of Psychosis Symptom Severity.) Note: Without this severity specifier, schizoaffective illness can be identified.

Note: to discover greater about Development and Course (factors which may be associated with age). See the corresponding sections in schizophrenia, bipolar I and II problems, and critical depressive contamination in their respective chapters for Risk and Prognostic Factors (environmental risk factors), Culture-Related Diagnostic Issues, and Gender-Related Diagnostic Issues.

DIAGNOSTIC CHARACTERISTICS

The assessment of an uninterrupted length of contamination within the course of which the affected person continues to show off lively or residual psychotic infection signs and symptoms and signs and symptoms and signs and symptoms serves as the premise for the prognosis of schizoaffective sickness. Usually, however no longer continuously, the psychotic infection is whilst the analysis is made. During the direction of the time. For schizophrenia, criterion A want to be happy. Models B (social brokenness) and F (prohibition of mental imbalance range jumble or different communication hassle of younger life beginning) for schizophrenia don't want to be met. There is a chief mood episode (main depressive or manic) that meets Criteria A for schizoaffective disorder similarly to assembly Criteria A for schizophrenia. Criterion A for schizoaffective sickness requires the most depressive episode to encompass pervasive depressed mood (the presence of markedly dwindled interest or satisfaction is not sufficient); that is because of the superiority of loss of interest or pride in schizophrenia. After Criterion A has been happy (Criterion C for schizoaffective sickness), the bulk of the illness's period is marked through episodes of melancholy or mania. Delusions or hallucinations need to final for at least weeks with out a high temper episode (depressive or manic) in the end in the course of the infection's lifetime in order to distinguish schizoaffective disorder from bipolar sickness or despair with psychotic abilties (Criterion B for schizoaffective disorder). (Criterion D for schizoaffective ailment) The effects of a substance or every exclusive medical scenario want to no longer be in charge for the signs and symptoms. For schizoaffective illness, criterion C stipulates that mood signs that meet the requirements for a high mood episode ought to be present for nearly all of the contamination's active and residual length. In comparison to the DSM-IV criterion, which most effective required an evaluation of the present day section of the contamination, criterion C requires an assessment of mood symptoms in some unspecified time inside the future of the path of a psychotic infection. The analysis is schizophrenia, not schizoaffective illness, if the mood signs last most effective a brief time. The clinician want to have a have a study the overall duration of the affected man or woman's psychotic contamination (i.E., both energetic and residual signs) and determine while considerable mood signs and signs and signs and symptoms (untreated or in want of remedy with antidepressant and/or temper-stabilizing medicine) determined the psychotic symptoms so one can determine whether or not or now not the affected individual's presentation meets Criterion C. Clinical judgment and sufficient historical records are required for this selection. For example, someone with schizophrenia who has had energetic and residual signs and symptoms and signs and symptoms for four years tales depressive and manic episodes that, taken together, last no a couple of yr in the 4 years of psychotic infection. Criterion C would possibly no longer be met through this presentation due to the reality, in addition to the five symptom domains indexed within the diagnostic requirements, the assessment of cognition, depression, and mania symptom domains is vital for distinguishing the diverse severa psychotic troubles and the schizophrenia spectrum.

In evaluation to schizophrenia, occupational functioning impairment isn't always a defining feature of the situation. Associated Features Supporting Diagnosis Schizoaffective ailment is associated with problems with self-care and restrained social contact, but horrible signs can be much less intense and much less continual than in schizophrenia. Poor perception, or annosognosia, is also commonplace in schizoaffective illness, however the deficits may be loads a great deal much less excessive and pervasive than in schizophrenia. If temper symptoms and signs persist after a remission of signs and symptoms meeting Criterion A for schizophrenia, humans with schizoaffective disease can be much more likely to boom episodes of vital depressive disorder or bipolar ailment. There might be associated liquor and specific substance-related messes. The analysis of schizoaffective illness cannot be aided through any herbal or diagnostic checks. It is unsure whether or now not structural or practical thoughts abnormalities, cognitive deficits, or genetic hazard factors distinguish schizoaffective ailment from schizophrenia.

Prevalence it might appear that schizoaffective sickness is set 1/three as commonplace as schizophrenia. Schizoaffective sickness is belief to have an effect on zero.Three percent of humans over their lifetime. Females have a higher incidence of schizoaffective disorder than adult males do, with the useful resource of and large because of the fact ladies have a higher prevalence of the depressive form.

Development and Course although onset can arise as early as teens or later in existence, the standard age of onset for schizoaffective sickness is early adulthood. When the pattern of temper episodes turns into extra obvious, a widespread wide variety of parents who've been first of all recognized with every distinct psychotic contamination will acquire the analysis of schizoaffective sickness. With the current-day diagnostic requirements, Criterion C, it is anticipated that a few human beings can be diagnosed with a disorder aside from schizoaffective ailment as their mood signs and signs and signs reduce. The evaluation for schizoaffective disease is worse than that for temper problems, but it is quite better than that for schizophrenia. There are many unique temporal styles in which schizophrenia can take area. One common pattern is as follows: A man or woman can also additionally moreover revel in persecutory and auditory hallucinations for 2 months previous to the onset of a extreme principal depressive episode. After that, the entire vital depressive episode and psychotic signs persist for 3 months. After that, the character without a doubt recovers from the precept depressive episode, however the psychotic signs and signs and symptoms final every specific month earlier than disappearing as nicely. Auditory hallucinations and delusions were present each in advance than and after the person's depressive segment during this era of contamination, and the person's signs simultaneously met requirements for a primary depressive episode and Criterion A for schizophrenia. The infection lasted approximately six months in overall, with psychotic symptoms on my own for the primary months, depressive and psychotic symptoms together for the next 3 months, and psychotic symptoms by myself for the final month. Due to the fact that the psychotic disturbance lasted longer than the depressive episode, the presentation warrants a schizoaffective sickness analysis on this situation.

Chapter 4: Chance And Prognostic Variables

Hereditary and physiological. First-degree family of schizophrenia sufferers may be much more likely to enlarge schizoaffective disease. People who have a first-degree relative with schizophrenia, bipolar sickness, or schizoaffective ailment can be much more likely to develop the disorder.

Culture-Related Diagnostic Issues When the affected person and the physician do not come from the identical cultural and economic ancient beyond, cultural and socioeconomic elements ought to be taken into consideration. In one life-style, beliefs that appear to be illogical, like witchcraft, may be widely held in every other. There is also some evidence inside the literature that African Americans and Hispanics are much more likely than different corporations to be diagnosed with both schizophrenia and schizoaffective disorder. Because of this, it is essential to take care to make sure that an assessment this is culturally appropriate takes into consideration each psychotic and affective symptoms.

Suicide Risk Factors the lifetime danger of suicide for humans with schizophrenia and schizoaffective sickness is 5%, and having depressive symptoms is related to a better threat of suicide. There is proof that the suicide expenses of human beings with schizophrenia or schizoaffective sickness in North America are higher than in European, Eastern European, South American, and Indian populations.

Functional Effects of Schizophrenia Schizoaffective disorder is associated with social and occupational sickness, however disease isn't a diagnostic criterion like it's far for schizophrenia, and there is lots of variation between people who've been diagnosed with the illness.

DIFFERENTIAL ANALYSIS

Other intellectual issues and illnesses. Psychotic and temper signs and symptoms and symptoms may be because of a huge style of highbrow fitness and clinical conditions, which have to be taken underneath attention within the differential diagnosis of schizoaffective illness. These consist of schizophrenia introduced on through manner of a unique medical situation; delirium; vital neurocognitive hassle; neurocognitive troubles or psychotic problems added on by using using manner of tablets or other drugs; intellectual ailments with bipolar signs and symptoms; intellectual contamination with psychotic developments; burdensome or bipolar issues with highbrow highlights; paranoid, schizotypal, or schizoid man or woman ailment; short-term psychosis; schizophrenic scenario; schizophrenia; illness of the thoughts; and exceptional psychotic troubles, every identified and unknown, as well as the schizophrenia spectrum. Psychotic and mood symptoms can be resulting from substance use and scientific conditions, so a psychotic sickness because of a few different medical scenario must be excluded. It may be tough to distinguish schizoaffective disorder from schizophrenia, despair, and bipolar issues with psychotic features. Criterion C is designed to distinguish among schizophrenia and schizoaffective infection, and Criterion B is designed to distinguish among schizoaffective disorder and a psychotic depressive or bipolar illness. More particularly, first-rate delusions and/or hallucinations lasting as a minimum two weeks with out a primary temper episode distinguish schizoaffective sickness from bipolar sickness or melancholy with psychotic features. Depressive or bipolar problems with psychotic capabilities, then again, have psychotic talents that generally seem in the path of the temper episode(s). The suitable evaluation can also trade from and to schizoaffective sickness due to the truth the ratio of temper to psychotic signs and symptoms and signs and symptoms and symptoms can trade through the years. For instance, if active psychotic or outstanding residual signs and signs and symptoms persist over severa years with out a recurrence of a temper episode, a evaluation of schizoaffective disease for a extreme and prominent essential depressive episode lasting 3 months at some degree within the primary six months of a chronic psychotic infection is probably modified to schizophrenia.

Mental contamination introduced on via each one of a kind scientific scenario. Because psychotic and mood signs and symptoms and symptoms can coexist with unique scientific conditions and substance use, psychotic disease can not be due to every distinct clinical state of affairs.

Disorders of schizophrenia, bipolar disease, and despair. It can be hard to differentiate schizoaffective illness from schizophrenia, depression, and bipolar problems with psychotic functions. Criterion C is designed to distinguish among schizophrenia and schizoaffective disorder, and Criterion B is designed to differentiate among schizoaffective ailment and a psychotic depressive or bipolar ailment. All the greater explicitly, schizoaffective turmoil may be recognized from a burdensome or bipolar hassle with maniacal elements in view of the presence of conspicuous fancies further to pipedreams for no lots plenty much less than approximately fourteen days without even a hint of a massive nation of thoughts episode. Depressive or bipolar ailment with psychotic features, as an alternative, commonly appear during the temper episode or episodes. The appropriate assessment may shift from and to schizoaffective illness because of fluctuations in the ratio of temper to psychotic symptoms and signs and symptoms over the years. For instance, if active psychotic or outstanding residual signs and symptoms and signs and symptoms persist over several years with out a recurrence of every other temper episode, a diagnosis of schizoaffective contamination for a extreme and distinguished crucial depressive episode lasting 3 months during the primary six months of a persistent psychotic contamination may be modified to schizophrenia.)

Comorbidity A lot of folks that are recognized with schizoaffective ailment additionally have other highbrow illnesses, specifically anxiety and substance use troubles. Additionally, the frequency of ailments is extended above base charge for anyone and turns on diminished destiny.

Diagnostic criteria for substance/clinical-added approximately psychotic sickness. The presence of 1 or both of the subsequent signs:

1. Delusions.

2. Hallucinations.

B. There is evidence from every (1) and (2)'s medical information, physical examination, or laboratory outcomes:

Criterion A's symptoms surfaced in the route of or fast after drug intoxication, withdrawal, or medicine exposure.

The disturbance isn't higher described through a psychotic ailment that is not as a result of the substance or remedy. The worried substance or medication can purpose the signs. The following are examples of such proof for an unbiased psychotic sickness:

The signs and symptoms and symptoms and symptoms commenced in advance than the substance or medication use started; After the acute withdrawal or severe intoxication has ended, the signs maintain for a enormous quantity of time (for instance, about one month): or rather there can be distinct evidence of a unfastened non-substance/medicinal drug incited insane turmoil (e.G., a past complete of repetitive non-substance/prescription associated episodes).

The disturbance doesn't truely seem whilst the man or woman is in delirium, The disturbance has a clinically massive impact on social, occupational, or different large regions of functioning misery or impairment.

Note: When Criterion A signs predominate in the clinical picture and whilst they may be sufficiently excessive to warrant medical interest, this evaluation must be made rather than substance intoxication or withdrawal.

Note for code: The desk beneath lists the ICD-9-CM and ICD-10-CIVI codes for the numerous substance or medication-introduced on psychotic problems. Keep in thoughts that the ICD-10-CM code for the equal substance beauty depends on whether or not or no longer or now not there may be a comorbid substance use illness. The clinician should report "moderate [substance] use illness" previous to the substance-prompted psychotic illness (e.G., "mild cocaine use sickness with cocaine-introduced approximately psychotic illness") if a slight substance use illness is comorbid with the substance-added about psychotic illness. The clinician should report either "slight [substance] use illness" or "excessive [substance] use disorder," counting on the severity of the comorbid substance use sickness, inside the fourth characteristic man or woman if a moderate or excessive substance use illness is comorbid with the substance-delivered about psychotic illness. The clinician want to satisfactory document the substance-brought about psychotic sickness if there may be no comorbid substance use illness (as an example, following a one-time heavy use of the substance).

Alcohol 291.Nine F10.159 FI zero.259 FI 0.959

Cannabis 292.Nine F12.159 FI 2.259 FI 2.959

Phencyclidine 292.Nine F16.159 FI 6.259 FI 6.959

Other hallucinogen 292.Nine FI 6.159 FI 6.259 FI 6.959

Inhalant 292.Nine F18.159 FI eight.259 FI 8.959

Sedative, hypnotic, or anxiolytic 292.Nine FI three.159

Beginning even as intoxicated: Assuming the guidelines are met for inebriation with the substance and the side results create in the direction of inebriation. Beginning at some point of withdrawal: If the conditions for substance withdrawal are met and withdrawal signs and signs and symptoms appear inside the course of or unexpectedly after the method. Please specify the severity in the interim: A quantitative evaluation of the primary signs and signs of psychosis—delusions, hallucinations, uncommon psychomotor conduct, and horrible symptoms and symptoms and signs and symptoms—is used to decide severity. On a 5-component scale that stages from zero (no longer gift) to 4 (present and excessive), every of these symptoms can be rated consistent with its modern severity (maximum extreme within the final seven days). In the bankruptcy titled "Assessment Measures," you may find out Clinician-Rated Dimensions of Psychosis Symptom Severity.) Note: Finding of substance/drug triggered crazy confusion may be made with out the usage of this seriousness specifier.

ICD-nine-CM Recording Procedures The specific substance (as an example, cocaine or dexamethasone) this is belief to be causing the delusions or hallucinations is wherein the call of the situation called substance/remedy-delivered about psychotic disease comes from. Based on the drug beauty, the table in the standards set is used to pick the diagnostic code. For substances that don't squeeze into any of the instructions (e.G., dexamethasone), the code for "remarkable substance" need to be applied; the time period "unknown substance" should be used at the same time as a substance is considered to be an etiological element but its precise elegance is unknown. The onset is extraordinary after the sickness's call (for example, onset in some unspecified time in the future of intoxication or withdrawal). ICD-nine-CM assigns a separate diagnostic code to the substance use illness, in evaluation to the recording techniques for ICD-IO-CM, which combine the substance-induced infection and the substance use ailment right into a single code. For instance, 292.Nine cocaine-precipitated psychotic disease with onset throughout intoxication is the analysis for someone with a extreme cocaine use illness who research delusions whilst intoxicated. Additionally, a excessive cocaine use sickness diagnosis of 304.20 is made. Each substance have to be indexed one after the other whilst more than one substances are belief to play a giant role within the onset of psychotic signs and symptoms (e.G., 292.Nine cannabis-brought on psychotic illness with onset in the course of intoxication, with intense cannabis use illness; 292.Nine slight phencyclidine use disease and phencyclidine-caused psychotic sickness that began out at the equal time as intoxicated). ICD-10-CM. The unique substance (as an instance, cocaine or dexamethasone) that is concept to be causing the delusions or hallucinations is in which the name of the state of affairs known as substance/remedy-introduced approximately psychotic disorder comes from. The demonstrative code is selected from the desk remembered for the requirements set, which relies upon on the drugs beauty and presence or nonattendance of a comorbid substance use jumble. For materials that don't squeeze into any of the instructions (e.G., dexamethasone), the code for "fantastic substance" with out a comorbid substance use should be completed; the class "unknown substance" without comorbid substance use ought to be used at the same time as a substance is considered to be an etiological detail however its particular elegance is unknown. While recording the call of the problem, the comorbid substance use jumble (if any) is recorded first, trailed by way of way of "with," trailed with the useful resource of manner of the call of the substance-initiated insane confusion, trailed with the aid of using the element of beginning (i.E., starting in the course of inebriation, starting during withdrawal). For example, the analysis for a person with excessive cocaine use sickness who critiques delusions at the same time as intoxicated is F14.259 immoderate cocaine use ailment with cocaine-induced psychotic disorder onset on the equal time as intoxicated. The comorbid excessive cocaine use disease isn't always given a separate diagnosis. If the substance-introduced on psychotic illness takes vicinity with out a comorbid substance use ailment (for example, following a one-time, heavy use of the substance), there can be no evidence of a comorbid substance use sickness (for instance, F16.959 phencyclidine-added approximately psychotic disease that starts offevolved whilst the man or woman is intoxicated). Each substance need to be indexed one after the opposite whilst a couple of materials are perception to play a huge role in the onset of psychotic signs and symptoms and symptoms and signs and symptoms and signs (for example, F12.259 severe hashish use ailment with cannabis-induced psychotic sickness; Phencyclidine-precipitated psychotic sickness with an onset in some unspecified time in the future of intoxication (F16.159 moderate phencyclidine use illness).

Diagnostic Characteristics Prominent delusions and/or hallucinations (Criterion A) which is probably idea to be due to the physiological effects of a substance or remedy (i.E., a drug of abuse, a remedy, or an exposure to a toxins) are the primary traits of substance/medicinal drug-induced psychotic sickness (Criterion B). Hallucinations that the individual realizes are because of drugs or remedy are not included in this magnificence; as an opportunity, they would be classified as substance intoxication or withdrawal with the accompanying qualifier "with perceptual disturbances" (this is applicable to alcohol withdrawal; consumption of cannabis; withdrawal that is sedative, hypnotic, or annoying; and intoxication with stimulants). The onset, direction, and one in all a type tendencies of a substance/remedy-introduced about psychotic illness distinguish it from a primary psychotic disease. There need to be proof of substance use, intoxication, or withdrawal from the beyond, physical exam, or laboratory outcomes for capsules of abuse. While number one psychotic troubles may also moreover begin preceding to the onset of substance/remedy use or can also moreover stand up within the course of periods of sustained abstinence, substance/treatment-added on psychotic problems show up at some point of or suddenly after publicity to a medication or after substance intoxication or withdrawal and may final for weeks. Psychotic signs and symptoms and signs and symptoms also can persist so long as the use of medicine or wonderful drug treatments continues after they are initiated. The presence of weird characteristics of a number one psychotic sickness (collectively with an top notch age at onset or path) is some different element to remember. For example, the onset of recent delusions in a 35-one year-vintage individual with out a earlier statistics of a number one psychotic disorder need to advise the presence of a substance or medicine-triggered psychotic illness. A substance or medication-brought about psychotic ailment can although rise up, irrespective of a records of number one psychotic issues. Interestingly, elements that recommend that the insane issue consequences are higher represented by using the use of an critical loopy problem incorporate industriousness of maniacal facet consequences for a large time-body (i.E., a month or extra) after the cease of substance inebriation or extreme substance withdrawal or after discontinuance of drugs use; or a records of primary psychotic problems that recur within the beyond. Because substance use troubles are not unusual amongst humans with non-substance/medication-introduced approximately psychotic troubles, exclusive reasons of psychotic signs and signs and symptoms need to be considered despite the fact that a person is intoxicated or retreating from tablets. For making crucial variations most of the various schizophrenia spectrum troubles and extraordinary psychotic problems, the assessment of cognition, depression, and mania symptom domains is important similarly to the 4 symptom area regions recognized within the diagnostic criteria.

Associated Signs and Symptoms That Support the Diagnosis Psychotic issues may be because of being intoxicated with the following materials: alcohol; hashish; hallucinogens, which incorporates phencyclidine and its derivatives; inhalants; anxiolytics, hypnotics, and sedatives; stimulants, which consist of cocaine; and extra materials, both recounted or unknown. Withdrawal from the subsequent substances may be related to psychotic troubles: alcohol; anxiolytics, hypnotics, and sedatives; and in addition materials, every recognized or unknown. A a part of the prescriptions responded to bring out insane thing effects contain sedatives and analgesics, anticholinergic specialists, anticonvulsants, hypersensitivity meds, antihypertensive and cardiovascular capsules, antimicrobial meds, antiparkinsonian meds, chemotherapeutic experts (e.G., cyclosporine, procarbazine), corticosteroids, gastrointestinal meds, muscle relaxants, nonsteroidal mitigating meds, specific non-prescription meds (e.G., phenylephrine, pseudoephedrine), energizer treatment, and disulfiram. Anticholinesterase, organophosphate insecticides, sarin and different nerve gases, carbon monoxide, carbon dioxide, and risky substances like gasoline or paint are the numerous pollution that have been related to psychotic signs and symptoms and symptoms and symptoms and signs.

Prevalence it is not mentioned how normal substance or remedy-brought about psychotic illness is amongst the general population. Substance/remedy-caused psychotic ailment is idea to have an impact on amongst 7% and 25% of folks that enjoy their first psychotic episode in one in each of a kind settings.

Development and Course The substance can also need to have a big effect on how the infection begins. In assessment to immoderate-dose alcohol or sedative use, which may additionally moreover take days or in all likelihood weeks to purpose psychosis, immoderate-dose cocaine smoking can cause psychosis in a remember of mins. In people with slight to excessive alcohol use illness, alcohol-precipitated psychotic sickness with hallucinations usually tremendous takes location after extended, heavy alcohol intake. The hallucinations are usually auditory. The medical trends of psychotic issues because of cocaine and amphetamine are similar. Amphetamine or some specific sympathomimetic with similar consequences can rapid purpose persecutory delusions. Formication, a hallucination of bugs or unique vermin crawling in or below the pores and pores and pores and skin, can bring about large pores and skin excoriations and scratching. Persecutory delusions, marked anxiety, emotional lability, and depersonalization are ordinary signs and symptoms and signs of cannabis-caused psychotic disorder, which can arise hastily after excessive-dose cannabis use. The condition usually goes away after a day, however it may final for a few days in some instances. When the offending agent is removed, substance/treatment-prompted psychotic disorder can also now and again persist, making it difficult to to start with distinguish it from an unbiased psychotic sickness. It has been stated that tablets like cocaine, amphetamines, and phencyclidine can reason brief psychosis which can ultimate for weeks or longer even after the drug is stopped and neuroleptic medicinal drug is used to cope with it. Polypharmacy and exposure to drug treatments for Parkinsonism, cardiovascular ailment, and unique clinical conditions also can boom the threat of psychosis in later existence, in preference to substance abuse, as a result of prescription medicinal drugs.

The presence of a stage that is consistent with toxicity might also moreover increase diagnostic reality for substances for which applicable blood levels are to be had (as an example, blood alcohol degree or different quantifiable blood levels like digoxin).

Functional Consequences of Substance/Medication-Induced Psychotic Disorder Substance/Medication-added approximately psychotic sickness is usually extraordinarily disabling, and as a cease end result, it takes area most usually in emergency rooms due to the fact humans frequently are on the lookout for remedy in the extreme care putting. However, in most cases, the incapacity is self-confined and disappears while the offending birthday party is removed.

Differential Diagnosis Intoxication or withdrawal from a substance Alternate perceptions that they apprehend as drug consequences can also stand up inside the ones intoxicated with stimulants, cannabis, the opioid meperidine or phencyclidine, or the ones taking flight from alcohol or sedatives. The evaluation isn't substance/medication-induced psychotic ailment if truth finding out for the ones tales stays intact (i.E., the man or woman recognizes that the perception is caused through substance use however neither believes in nor acts on it). Instead, a prognosis of substance intoxication or withdrawal with perceptual disturbances (which incorporates cocaine intoxication with perceptual disturbances) is made. Hallucinogen persisting notion illness is the time period used to provide an explanation for "flashback" hallucinations, that would maintain lengthy after the individual has stopped using hallucinogens. The psychotic symptoms are taken into consideration to be an associated function of the delirium and are not recognized one by one in the event that they stand up totally during the course of a delirium, which include in immoderate alcohol withdrawal. Major or slight neurocognitive disorder with behavioral disturbance is the diagnosis for delusions in the context of a number one or slight neurocognitive infection.

Mental contamination brought on by using some different medical scenario. A substance or medicine-prompted psychotic infection due to a prescribed remedy for a intellectual or scientific situation need to begin at the identical time as the man or woman is taking the drugs (or even as they're withdrawing from it, if the drugs has a withdrawal syndrome). The clinician must preserve in thoughts the possibility that the psychotic symptoms and symptoms are because of the physiological effects of the medical scenario in area of the medicine due to the truth humans with scientific situations regularly take medicinal capsules for the ones conditions. In this situation, psychotic sickness due to a few different medical state of affairs is diagnosed. For this kind of judgment, the information frequently serves due to the fact the number one foundation. To empirically decide for that character whether or not or no longer the medicine is the causative agent, every now and then a exchange inside the treatment for the scientific condition—along with remedy substitution or discontinuation—may be required.

Both diagnoses—i.E., psychotic disease due to any other clinical situation and substance/treatment-added on psychotic illness—can be given if the clinician has determined that the disturbance is on account of every a medical condition and the use of medicine or one of a kind drugs.

Diagnostic Criteria A: Prominent hallucinations or delusions due to a highbrow infection B. The disturbance is the direct pathophysiological very last outcomes of each other clinical situation, as confirmed via way of the data, physical exam, or laboratory results. C. An extra intellectual infection cannot higher offer an reason behind the disturbance. D. The disturbance doesn't actually rise up at the equal time as the man or woman is in delirium. E. The disturbance has a clinically sizeable impact on social, occupational, or unique extremely good areas of functioning distress or impairment.

Note for code: The highbrow infection's name must consist of the name of the alternative scientific circumstance (as an example, 293.Eighty one [F06.2] psychotic illness because of malignant lung neoplasm, with delusions). Due to the medical state of affairs, the alternative situation should be coded and listed one after the opposite preceding to the psychotic illness (as an instance, 162.Nine [C34.90] malignant lung neoplasm; 293.Eighty one [F06.2] psychotic sickness with delusions due to a malignant lung neoplasm).

Please specify the severity within the propose time: A quantitative evaluation of the primary signs of psychosis—delusions, hallucinations, incredible psychomotor conduct, and terrible signs and symptoms and signs and symptoms—is used to determine severity. On a 5-issue scale that stages from zero (not gift) to 4 (present and severe), every of those signs and symptoms may be rated regular with its modern-day-day severity (most severe within the last seven days). In the monetary disaster titled "Assessment Measures," you could locate Clinician-Rated Dimensions of Psychosis Symptom Severity.) Note: It is viable to make a analysis of psychotic sickness primarily based on each different scientific situation with out making use of this severity specifier.

Specifiers the assessment of cognition, despair, and mania symptom domain names is essential for making vital differences maximum of the numerous schizophrenia spectrum troubles and extraordinary psychotic troubles in addition to the symptom area regions identified inside the diagnostic requirements.

Diagnostic Characteristics Prominent delusions or hallucinations which may be deemed to be because of the physiological consequences of some other clinical situation and are not better described by way of every other highbrow ailment are vital characteristics of psychotic contamination due to a few different medical condition. For instance, the symptoms and signs and signs and signs and symptoms are not a psychologically mediated reaction to a intense scientific scenario, wherein case a analysis of short psychotic contamination with marked stressor would be suitable.

Chapter 5: The Most Diagnostic

Reality that the delusions or hallucinations are due to a scientific state of affairs is supplied with the aid of the use of the temporal affiliation of the onset or exacerbation of the state of affairs. Associated Features Supporting Diagnosis Treatments for the underlying condition that independently growth the risk of psychosis, which incorporates steroids for autoimmune troubles, can also be contributing elements.

Due to the splendid fashion of underlying scientific etiologies, it's miles hard to estimate the superiority prices of psychotic disease because of a few different clinical situation. The predicted lifetime prevalence levels from 0.21 percent to zero.Fifty four%. When the prevalence information are damaged down thru age organization, human beings over 65 have a far higher prevalence of zero.Seventy 4 percentage than human beings in younger age groups.

In addition, fees of psychosis variety based on the underlying clinical scenario; Untreated metabolic and endocrine troubles, autoimmune issues like systemic lupus erythematosus and N-methyl-D-aspartate receptor autoimmune encephalitis, and temporal lobe epilepsy are the most customarily related to psychosis. The epileptic psychosis has been further divided into interictal, postictal, and ictal psychosis. Postictal psychosis, which affects among 2% and seven.Eight% of epileptics, is the maximum common of these. Females may also additionally have a better prevalence of the sickness in older people, however one in every of a type gender-related tendencies are unsure and variety substantially with the distributions of the underlying clinical situations.

Development and Course a psychotic infection that is due to a few distinctive scientific state of affairs can be a single, brief episode or a recurrent situation that cycles through exacerbations and remissions of the underlying situation. Psychotic signs and symptoms can also persist extended after a medical occasion (together with a psychotic contamination on account of a focal thoughts damage), irrespective of the truth that treating the underlying clinical state of affairs commonly resolves the psychosis. The psychosis may additionally moreover furthermore have a protracted-term course in persistent situations like a couple of sclerosis or epilepsy with persistent interictal psychosis. The phenomenology of psychotic sickness due to a few special scientific scenario does no longer substantially range with age at onset. However, the disorder is greater large in older age businesses, most possibly because of the developing scientific burden associated with advanced age and the cumulative results of risky exposures and age-related strategies (which include atherosclerosis). The underlying medical conditions are probably to exchange through the years; more youthful age corporations are more likely to be laid low with epilepsy, head trauma, autoimmune sicknesses, and neoplastic sicknesses of early to midlife, at the same time as older age groups are more likely to be affected by stroke illness, anoxic sports, and more than one device comorbidities. Preexisting cognitive, imaginative and prescient, and paying attention to impairments, similarly to different underlying factors like age, can also enhance the chance of psychosis, in all likelihood via lowering the edge at which psychosis can stand up.

Modifiers to the direction are danger and prognostic elements. The most widespread have an impact on on route is the identity and remedy of the underlying clinical circumstance, notwithstanding the fact that preexisting injuries to the crucial annoying tool (together with head trauma and cerebrovascular infection) also can bring about a worse course final outcomes.

The diagnostic exams used to diagnose psychotic ailment due to each different medical situation will variety counting on the person's clinical situation. Psychotic symptoms and symptoms and signs and symptoms can be added on via the use of a large fashion of medical situations. Neurological conditions like tumors, cerebrovascular ailment, Huntington's sickness, more than one sclerosis, epilepsy, deafness, migraine, and infections of the crucial involved tool are examples of these. Endocrine conditions like hyper- and hypothyroidism, hyper- and hypoparathyroidism, hyper- and hypoadrenocorticism, metabolic situations like hypoxia, hypercarbia, and hypoglycemia, fluid or electrolyte imbalances, illnesses of the liver or the etiological clinical scenario is pondered in the findings of the bodily exam, laboratory consequences, and kinds of incidence or onset.

Despite the reality that superb conditions like epilepsy and more than one sclerosis are related to prolonged expenses of suicide, which can be further increased inside the presence of psychosis, suicide danger inside the context of psychotic disease because of every different scientific condition isn't in truth defined.

Functional Disabilities of a Psychotic Disorder Caused via the use of the usage of a Medical Condition Functional incapacity is generally excessive within the context of a psychotic disorder because of a systematic situation. However, it could be very superb relying on the form of circumstance, and it is probable to get better if the situation is efficaciously handled.

Delirium due to differential analysis. Delirium is frequently determined thru hallucinations and delusions; but, if the disturbance best occurs within the direction of a delirium, a separate analysis of psychotic ailment due to every specific scientific condition isn't always made. Major or mild neurocognitive infection with behavioral disturbance is the diagnosis for delusions within the context of a prime or slight neurocognitive disease. Psychotic sickness delivered on with the aid of medicine or different pills. A substance/medicine-precipitated psychotic sickness have to be taken into consideration if there is evidence of latest or extended substance use (in conjunction with medicines with psychoactive effects), withdrawal from a substance, or publicity to a pollution (collectively with LSD [lysergic acid diethylamide] intoxication, alcohol withdrawal, and so forth.). Depending on the person, length, or amount of the substance used, signs and symptoms that stand up in the course of or quick after (i.E., within four weeks) substance intoxication, withdrawal, or treatment use may be mainly indicative of a substance-introduced approximately psychotic illness. Both psychotic ailment because of every exceptional clinical scenario and substance/medicinal drug-introduced on psychotic disorder can be given if the clinician has determined that the disturbance is because of each substance use and a clinical condition. Crazy turmoil. A psychotic ailment because of a scientific state of affairs should be distinguished from a psychotic illness with psychotic capabilities, which encompass schizophrenia, delusional sickness, or schizoaffective illness. No precise and direct physiological mechanisms which is probably associated with a systematic situation can be examined in psychotic problems, depressive troubles, or bipolar issues with psychotic functions. The need for a complete evaluation to rule out the evaluation of psychotic disorder because of each other clinical situation is generally advocated thru the late age at onset and the absence of a non-public or circle of relatives records of schizophrenia or delusional disorder. Due to a systematic state of affairs, auditory hallucinations in which voices talk complicated sentences are greater everyday of schizophrenia than of psychotic sickness. Other varieties of hallucinations, like visual and olfactory ones, frequently factor to a psychotic illness introduced on by way of the use of some distinct clinical situation or through pills or specific medicinal pills.

Comorbidity Psychotic disorder due to every exceptional scientific scenario is related to concurrent important neurocognitive illness (dementia) in human beings over eighty.

The man or woman has at the least one manic episode that meets the standards (Criteria A-D below "Manic Episode" above) and the cultural norms for the manner to precise distress within the context of loss. This preference will necessarily necessitate the utility of scientific judgment. B. The occasion of the hyper and massive burdensome episode(s) isn't higher made feel of through the usage of schizoaffective confusion, schizophrenia, schizophreniform jumble, whimsical turmoil, or unique determined or indistinct schizophrenia range and awesome maniacal hassle.

Procedures for Coding and Recording The form of modern-day or maximum extremely-present day episode and its severity, presence of psychotic abilties, and remission reputation decide the diagnostic code for bipolar I illness. Only if all of the criteria for a manic or primary depressive episode are currently met are current severity and psychotic capabilities indicated. Remission specifiers are best encouraged at the same time as a manic, hypomanic, or maximum important depressive episode does now not currently meet all of the requirements. These are the codes:

Bipolar 1 illness Current or most ultra-modern episode manic Current or maximum cutting-edge episode hypomanic Current or most current episode depressed Current or maximum contemporary episode unspecified.

The so-known as pangs of grief are waves of dysphoria that typically subside over the path of a few days to weeks. These waves commonly deliver up memories or thoughts of the deceased. A MDE's depressed mood lasts longer and is unrelated to unique mind or problems. The aggravation of melancholy might be joined via manner of sure feelings and humor which are ordinary of the unavoidable despondency and hopelessness normal for a big burdensome episode.

Instead of the self-essential or pessimistic ruminations of a MDE, the concept content fabric fabric related to grief commonly capabilities a preoccupation with mind and reminiscences of the deceased. While in a MDE, feelings of worthlessness and self-loathing are not unusual, conceitedness is usually maintained in grief. Grief-related self-doubt usually revolves spherical perceived shortcomings with the deceased (which consist of no longer travelling them sufficient or telling them how a whole lot they have been cherished). In a number one depressive episode, such mind are targeted on completing one's non-public lifestyles because of feeling worthless, not worthy of life, or unable to cope with the ache of melancholy. When a bereaved person thinks approximately loss of lifestyles and absence of life, those mind are commonly targeted at the deceased and in all likelihood about "becoming a member of" the deceased.

Seriousness and loopy specifiers don't depend huge range; cases that are not in remission are coded 296.Forty (F31.Zero). There aren't any severity, psychotic, or remission standards. Code 296.7 (F31.Nine). *** Regardless of the severity of the episode, code the code "with psychotic functions" if psychotic talents are gift. The following terms need to be listed in the order that they seem in a analysis's name: bipolar I disorder, the form of present day or most state-of-the-art episode, the severity, psychotic, or remission criteria, and as many specific requirements without codes as are applicable to the present day-day or maximum present day episode.

Diagnostic Features A first-rate length of abnormally multiplied, expansive, or irritable temper and constantly prolonged interest or energy this is gift for maximum of the day, nearly every day, for at least one week (or any length if hospitalization is crucial) with at the least 3 more symptoms and signs and symptoms from Criterion B. If the mood is irritable in choice to expanded or expansive, at the least four Criterion B symptoms want to be present. A manic episode's mood is frequently referred to as euphoric, excessively thrilled, excessive, or "feeling on pinnacle of the sector." The mood can be characterized via an limitless and haphazard enthusiasm for interpersonal, sexual, or place of job interactions in some times because it is so infectious. For example, the man or woman might start prolonged conversations with strangers in public on their private. When a person is denied their desires or has been the use of substances, the vital mood is often irritable in preference to stepped forward. Liability (moreover referred to as the alternation amongst euphoria, dysphoria, and irritability) refers to speedy temper adjustments that could arise over quick intervals of time. In kids, bliss, unreasonableness and "silliness" are commonplace nearly approximately particular activities; but, these signs and symptoms and symptoms and symptoms might also moreover meet Criterion A if they will be recurrent, irrelevant for the state of affairs, and above the child's ordinary developmental degree. If the kid's happiness is unusual (i.E., precise from baseline) and the mood alternate coincides with signs and symptoms and signs and symptoms that meet Criterion B for mania, diagnostic reality is extended; However, parents that are acquainted with the child need to take a look at constantly extended ranges of hobby or energy alongside component the trade in temper. The man or woman might also additionally address more than one new initiatives that overlap at some stage in the manic segment. The duties are frequently commenced with the resource of using people who don't recognize a good deal about the undertaking, and now not anything seems out of attain. It's feasible that the stepped forward interest stages will display up at strange hours of the day. According to Criteria B1, inflated vanity can range from uncritical self-self belief to marked grandiosity or even attain delusional proportions. The individual can also moreover tackle complicated responsibilities like writing a unique or seeing exposure for an impractical invention however having no particular abilties or revel in. Common are grandiose delusions, which embody the notion that one has a special connection to a well-known individual. It is everyday for youngsters to overestimate their talents and consider that they are the exceptional at a endeavor or the first-rate child inside the beauty; However, the grandiosity criterion ought to be taken into consideration satisfied whilst such beliefs are present no matter easy evidence to the other, or when the child tries feats which can be sincerely risky and, most importantly, constitute a exchange from the child's ordinary behavior. One of the most famous highlights is a dwindled requirement for relaxation (Model B2) and is unique from sleep deprivation wherein the singular desires to relaxation or wants to rest however can't. The individual would in all likelihood relaxation a piece, if thru any technique, or can also stir some hours earlier than expected, feeling refreshed and ready for industrial business enterprise. When the sleep disturbance is immoderate, the character may not experience tired even after going days without drowsing. A manic episode typically starts even as sleepiness decreases. (Criterion B3), speech can be rapid, compelled, loud, and difficult to break. It is possible for humans to speak constantly without thinking about what brilliant people want to mention, regularly in an intrusive way or with out thinking about how crucial what is stated is. Jokes, puns, funny irrelevancies, theatricality, dramatic gestures, making a song, and excessive gesturing are all traits of speech. Clamor and forcefulness of discourse regularly become more amazing than what's conveyed. Speech can be marked through using complaints, adverse remarks, or angry tirades if the man or woman's temper is greater irritable than expansive, especially if tries are made to interrupt the individual. Criterion A and Criterion B symptoms can be decided by using the usage of manner of depressive symptoms and symptoms and signs. (Criterion B4) Frequently, the character's mind race at a charge quicker than they will be expressed verbally. A almost non-prevent go together with the glide of fast speech with abrupt shifts from one problem to some other often demonstrates a flight of thoughts. Speech can end up disorganized, incoherent, and specially distressing whilst there may be excessive flight of thoughts. Sometimes it's tough to talk because of the reality one's mind are so crowded.

Concerns (Criterion B7) without having the coins to pay for them, the person might also purchase a number of useless subjects and from time to time provide them away. Sexual conduct can take the shape of infidelity or random sexual encounters with strangers, often without considering the possibility of sexually transmitted illnesses or the outcomes on relationships. To save you harm to oneself or others (e.G., economic losses, unlawful sports activities activities, loss of employment, self-injurious behavior), the manic episode need to purpose a huge impairment in social or occupational functioning or necessitate hospitalization. Manic signs and symptoms or syndromes which may be due to the physiological consequences of a drug of abuse (e.G., in the context of cocaine or amphetamine intoxication), the element outcomes of medicinal capsules or treatments (e.G., steroids, L-dopa, antidepressants, stimulants), or some different medical scenario do now not depend number toward the evaluation of bipolar I sickness. By definition, the presence of psychotic competencies at some point of a manic episode moreover satisfies Criterion C. However, enough proof for a manic episode diagnosis (Criterion D) is a completely syndromal manic episode that takes place at some stage in treatment (e.G., medicinal capsules, electroconvulsive treatment, slight remedy) or drug use and lasts past the physiological effect of the inducing agent (i.E., after a remedy has absolutely left the individual's tool or the outcomes of electroconvulsive treatment can be expected to have dissipated). One or signs—especially accelerated irritability, edginess, or agitation following antidepressant use—ought to not be taken as conclusive for the diagnosis of a manic or hypomanic episode or a bipolar disorder analysis. To be identified with bipolar I illness, you have to have a manic episode, but you don't have to have hypomania or important depressive episodes. However, they might stand up previous to or after a manic episode. The textual content for bipolar II sickness gives complete descriptions of the diagnostic functions of a hypomanie episode, and the textual content for crucial depressive illness offers entire descriptions of the diagnostic functions of a prime depressive episode.

Associated Signs and Symptoms That Support a Manic Episode During a manic episode, human beings frequently fail to understand that they'll be ill or in need of remedy and vehemently withstand tries to get hold of treatment. Individuals can also adopt a more sexually suggestive or flamboyant style for his or her clothing, makeup, or personal look. A sharper sense of heady scent, being attentive to, or imaginative and prescient is professional through some. The manic episode may be positioned with the resource of playing and delinquent behaviors. When delusional, some humans may also turn out to be bodily violent or suicidal, in addition to end up adverse and bodily threatening to others. Poor judgment, loss of perception, and hyperactivity regularly bring about catastrophic outcomes of a manic episode, which includes involuntary hospitalization, criminal problems, and immoderate economic troubles. State of mind may additionally pass brief to outrage or wretchedness. During a manic episode, depressive signs can rise up and ultimate for minutes, hours, or, a whole lot much less regularly, days (see "with combined skills" specifier, pages).

Prevalence According to the DSM-IV, the 12-month occurrence estimate for bipolar I sickness in the continental United States turn out to be 0.6%. In eleven countries, the 12-month occurrence of bipolar I contamination ranged from 0% to 6%. The lifetime prevalence ratio of fellows to women is ready 1.1:1.

Chapter 6: What Is Schizophrenia?

Schizophrenia is a critical highbrow infection in which the character translates truth abnormally. This situation can result in a mixture of hallucinations, disorganized thinking and conduct that preclude and disable the every day functioning of the individual.

People with schizophrenia require lifelong remedy. Early remedy facilitates preserve signs under control earlier than extreme complications boom and allows to have a higher long-time period outlook.

Symptoms

Schizophrenia impacts a person's wondering, emotions, and behavior. Symptoms can vary but normally delusions, hallucinations, disorganized speech and absence of capability to function are present. Symptoms also can moreover the following:

. Delusions- This is described as fake ideals, not based totally on fact. For example, they assume they will be being persecuted to damage them; they have conversations with themselves; they think they may be a well-known individual; that someone is in love with them; that a tragedy is ready to reveal up. The delusions are located in almost absolutely all people with schizophrenia.

. Hallucinations- This consists of taking note of or seeing matters that aren't there or aren't actual. But, the person with schizophrenia perceives it as a real truth notwithstanding being tested otherwise. Hallucinations can rise up in any of your senses, however listening to voices is the maximum not unusual.

. Disorganized mind- their thoughts stand up disorganized speech. Effective verbal exchange is tough, solutions to questions can be in part or unrelated. Rarely, their speech also can include putting unrelated or nonsensical terms collectively, moreover called phrase salad.

. Extreme disorganization or abnormal conduct and motion- This can display up itself in a number of methods, from childlike behavior to unpredictable agitation. His behavior isn't always centered on a aim, making it hard for him to complete obligations. Their behavior may moreover consist of resistance to recommendations, beside the factor posture, loss of reaction, or excessive or purposeless moves.

. Negative signs and symptoms- This refers to terrible or incapacity to feature commonly. For instance, the individual stops grooming, or appears unemotional (no eye touch, uses an uneventful voice). Also the character loses interest in sports activities of each day dwelling. Social isolation or disability to enjoy or enjoy pride.

Symptoms can range in type and severity through the years, with periods of worsening and remission. Some may be constantly present.

In guys, signs and symptoms and signs and symptoms of schizophrenia begin in the 20 to twenty-five age variety. It isn't always common for a kid to be diagnosed with schizophrenia and the assessment is uncommon in humans older than forty five years.

Symptoms in kids

The symptoms of schizophrenia in youngsters are much like the ones in adults, however the situation can be extra tough to understand. This is in element because of the truth the start of the signs and symptoms and symptoms of schizophrenia go to the fore with those of the same old improvement in formative years. Such as:.

. Withdrawal from buddies and family (social isolation).

. Poor usual performance in school.

. Sleep problems (insomnia).

. Irritability, despair.

. Lack of motivation.

Also, the usage of entertainment tablets, collectively with marijuana, methamphetamine, and LSD, can reason signs and symptoms much like those of schizophrenia. Compared to adults, teenagers

can.Less vulnerable to delusions.. More vulnerable to seen hallucinations.

When to look a doctor

People with schizophrenia nearly in no way comprehend that their problems are attributed to highbrow troubles that require clinical attention. It is sort of typically as plenty as the circle of relatives or family to are searching for for help from them.

If you determined that a person you understand may additionally moreover additionally have symptoms and signs of schizophrenia, discuss your problems. Although you cannot pressure someone to are searching out professional assist, you may offer help and encouragement to attempting to find help from an authorized professional or mental health professional.

If the individual poses a hazard of danger to himself or others. Also, if the character is not able to offer for themselves (their meals, clothing, or safe haven), you could want to name 911 or precise emergency assist to be evaluated through way of a intellectual fitness expert.

Chapter 7: Causes Of Schizophrenia

It is not recognized what reasons this condition, however professionals don't forget that the mixture of genetics, chemical imbalances inside the mind and the surrounding surroundings play a function inside the development of this situation.

Problems with fantastic natural mind chemical substances, along side neurotransmitters called dopamine and glutamate, can be humans to schizophrenia.

Images of the neurological tool display versions inside the systems of the thoughts and imperative worried tool in human beings with schizophrenia. Although experts aren't positive of the importance of those modifications, they propose that schizophrenia is a ailment of the thoughts.

Risks of tormented by schizophrenia.

Although an appropriate reason of schizophrenia is unknown, some elements appear increase the risk of developing this disorder,along with:

. Family information of schizophrenia.

. Some headaches in pregnancy or beginning, which consist of malnutrition, publicity to pollutants or viruses which could impact mind development.

. Taking drugs or drugs that adjust the thoughts (psychoactive or psychotropic) at some point of early life and in their younger years.

Chapter 8: Complications Of Schizophrenia

Without proper remedy, schizophrenia can bring about a excessive problem which can have an effect on all areas of his life. Complications of schizophrenia may also embody:

. Suicide, suicide try and mind of suicide.

. Anxiety and Obsessive Compulsive Disorder (OCD).

. Depression.

. Drug abuse, alcohol along with nicotine.

. Inability to paintings or attend college.

. Financial and steady haven troubles.

. Social isolation.

. Medical and health problems.

. Risk of being abused.

. Abusive conduct, although it is unusual.

Prevention

There isn't any sure manner to prevent schizophrenia, but following your treatment plan can save you a relapse or worsening of symptoms. Also, specialists are hopeful that learning more approximately the dangers and factors of getting schizophrenia can help early prognosis and treatment of the infection.

Chapter 9: Diagnosis

The evaluation of schizophrenia includes ruling out distinct highbrow illnesses and symptoms which are not because of drug remedies, drug use, and every other clinical situation.

The evaluation of schizophrenia may additionally moreover moreover consist of:

. Physical examination- This to rule out distinct issues that may be causing the problem or symptoms and signs and signs and symptoms and moreover to diagnose every other headaches.

. Testing- This to rule out some conditions which could cause comparable symptoms and symptoms and signs and signs and screening to check for alcohol and pills. The health practitioner may additionally additionally furthermore advocate have a study pics at the side of MRI or CT take a look at.

. Psychiatric assessment- A medical physician or highbrow fitness expert examines your intellectual fitness by means of the usage of way of looking your look, behavior, and questions about hallucinations, delusions, temperament, substance use, and the potential for suicide or violence. This moreover includes own family and personal records.

. Diagnostic Criteria for Schizophrenia

A medical doctor or highbrow health professional also can use the Criteria and Statistical Manual for Mental Disorders (DSM-five), published through manner of the American Psychiatric Association.

Chapter 10: Treatment

Schizophrenia illness requires lifelong remedy, no matter the reality that its signs and symptoms have reduced. Medication treatment and psychological treatment can assist manipulate the situation. In some times, it may require hospitalization.

A psychiatrist with revel in in treating schizophrenia commonly guides treatment. The treatment team can also include a psychologist, social employee, psychiatric nurse, and in all likelihood a case manager to coordinate care. This institution of specialists can be determined in clinics which might be experts in treating schizophrenia.

Medications

Medications are the primary remedy in schizophrenia. Antipsychotic medicinal tablets are the maximum common medicinal drugs advocated. They are believed to manipulate signs with the useful aid of affecting the mind's neurotransmitter dopamine.

The cause in treatment with antipsychotic medicinal capsules is to manipulate symptoms and signs and symptoms and signs with the lowest dose possible. The psychiatrist also can furthermore attempt several tablets, wonderful dosages, or combinations over the years till the preferred give up end result is finished. Other drugs which could assist are antidepressants and anti-anxiety. It may take severa weeks to look an development in symptoms.

Because a number of the medicine for schizophrenia can cause extreme facet results, people with schizophrenia occasionally refuse to take them. Depending at the cooperation of the character, the treatment and the medicine may be affected. For example, mother and father that do not want to take oral medicinal pills also can need medicinal tablets to take shipping of in injections alternatively.

Ask your medical doctor about the blessings and thing consequences of any medicinal drug prescribed.

Second technology antipsychotics

This new 2nd era antipsychotics are normally preferred because of the truth they have got a lower hazard of massive issue effects than the number one generation. Antipsychotics include the second technology.

. Aripiprazole (Abilify)

. Asenapine (Saphris)

. Brexpiprazole (Rexulti)

. Cariprazine (Vraylar)

. Clozapine (Clozaril, Versacloz)

. Iloperidone (Fanapt)

. Lurasidone (Latuda)

. Olanzapine (Zyprexa)

. Paliperidone (Invega)

. Quetiapine (Seroquel)

. Risperidone (Risperdal)

. Ziprasidone (Geodon)

First-technology antipsychotics

These antipsychotics have commonplace and doubtlessly severe factor consequences at the neurological gadget, together with the opportunity of growing movement troubles (tardive dyskinesia) which could or won't be reversible. The first era of antipsychotic Include:

. Chlorpromazine

. Fluphenazine

. Perphenazine

. Haloperidol

These antipsychotics are almost normally less costly than second generation antipsychotics, in particular the general variations, which may be an critical attention in prolonged-time period treatment.

Long-acting injectable antipsychotics

Some antipsychotics can be injected intramuscularly or subcutaneously. They are typically given each 2 to 4 weeks, counting on the drugs. Ask your medical doctor for greater statistics on injectable medicinal tablets. This may be an opportunity for humans who have hassle sticking to their treatment ordinary or for folks that prefer to take a whole lot a whole lot much less tablets or oral drug remedies.

These are a number of the injectable tablets:

. Aripiprazole (Abilify, Maintena, Aristada)

. Fluphenazine decanoate

. Haloperidol decanoate

. Paliperidone (Invega Sustena, Invega Trinza)

. Risperidone (Risperdal Consta, Perseris) Psychosocial

Intervention

When the psychosis catastrophe has advanced, psychology and psychosocial healing approaches are usually started out out. They might also encompass:

. Individual Therapy - Individual remedy can assist normalize thought styles. It additionally teaches a way to deal with stress and become aware about the preliminary signs and symptoms and symptoms and signs of a relapse. This can help the man or woman stricken by schizophrenia to manipulate their infection.

.Social capabilities training- This specializes in enhancing conversation and social interactions, in addition to the capability to take part in every day sports activities sports.

Family Therapy- This gives assist and education to the circle of relatives dealing with schizophrenia.

. Vocational and Employment Rehabilitation Support- This focuses on assisting the man or woman with schizophrenia prepare for employment, find out employment, and stay in their jobs.

Most human beings with schizophrenia require some shape of each day useful resource. Many businesses have programs to help them discover jobs, stable haven, self-help groups, and at some stage in crises. A case manager will let you locate the ones resources. With right treatment, most human beings with schizophrenia can manipulate their state of affairs.

Hospitalization

During periods of disaster or times with excessive signs and symptoms, hospitalization may be essential to make certain his safety, nutrients, desirable enough sleep, and clean hygiene.

Electroconvulsive Therapy

For adults who do not reply to medicinal pills, electroconvulsive remedy (ECT) may be taken into consideration. ECT can also help humans have despair.

Dealing with one of these intense intellectual sickness as schizophrenia can be difficult, each for the person with the scenario and for their own family and pals. Here are a few tips on the way to deal:.

Learning about schizophrenia- Education can assist the man or woman suffering with the situation to recognize the importance of following their treatment and preserving the plan of care. Education also can assist own family and buddies understand the scenario and have more compassion for the individual tormented by it.

. Focus on their goal: Managing schizophrenia in an ongoing gadget. Keeping treatment desires in thoughts can assist the character with schizophrenia live encouraged. Help the one which you love take duty for handling their scenario and jogging within the path in their desires.

. Avoid alcohol and drug use- The use of alcohol, nicotine or leisure pills might also need to make it difficult to address the contamination. If the only that you love has an addiction, quitting goes to be difficult. Seek help from the health crew within the fine way to address this trouble.

. Learn approximately social assist services- These offerings can help you discover low-price refuge, transportation, and different day by day sports activities.

. Learn about pressure manipulate and rest-People with the state of affairs and their loved ones can benefit from the ones pressure good buy remedies together with: yoga, or tai-chi.

. Join a useful resource institution - Support agencies for people with schizophrenia - In those corporations you can discover assist in people who've also or are going thru comparable conditions. Family help companies also can assist households and friends cope.

How to prepare for your appointment?

If you're searching for help for someone tormented by schizophrenia, you can begin thru the use of seeing his medical physician, however the fact that most of the time you may be proper away said his psychiatrist.

Chapter 11: How Are You Able To Prepare In Your Appointment?

To prepare to your appointment, create a listing consisting:

. Any symptoms the only that you love is experiencing. Including the ones unrelated to the reason in your appointment.

. Key information- Including any stresses the man or woman is going through/ important modifications of their lives.

Medications - Vitamins, Herbs, and different nutritional nutritional dietary supplements he's taking, together with dosages.

. Questions to the scientific physician

Take your beloved to the appointments. Getting information from his medical doctor will assist you recognize what he's dealing with and the approaches you could help him.

For people with schizophrenia Here are a few primary inquiries to ask your scientific medical health practitioner.

. What is the reason of the signs and signs?

. What may be considered one of a type motives of the signs and symptoms and symptoms and signs and symptoms and signs?

. What sorts of assessments does he need?

. Which is the outstanding remedy?

. What is the opportunity to the number one cautioned treatment approach?

. What is the top notch manner to help and assist him?

. Do you have got got were given written literature or pamphlets with fabric on the situation?

. What net websites do you suggest?

. What questions are you capable of assume from the medical doctor?

. What are the signs and symptoms, after I first be aware them?

. Does he have a family records of schizophrenia?

. Are the symptoms occasional or non-save you?

. How nicely does the best that you love function in his each day lifestyles? Does he wash each day? Is he attending school or art work?

. Has he been recognized with every one-of-a-kind situations?

What medicinal tablets are he currently taking?

Chapter 12: Myths And Facts Of Schizophrenia

Schizophrenia is a vital sickness that impacts how a person thinks, feels, and acts. People with schizophrenia have hassle distinguishing amongst what's real and what's imaginary.

Schizophrenia is not because of kids research, loss of proper parenting, or lack of energy of will.

Most people with schizophrenia aren't violent and do no longer reason chance to others.

Schizophrenia impacts 1% of the place's populace.

In the us, one in a hundred, 2.Five million, has this sickness. It does now not respect race, subculture or economic borders. Symptoms generally seem some of the a while of thirteen to twenty-five, but regularly seem earlier, more in men than women.

Symptoms that may be indicative of early signs of schizophrenia.

. Hearing or seeing things that are not there.

. A steady feeling that they're searching

. Body positions which might be unusual

. Feeling detached in very essential conditions

. Study or paintings impairment/incapacity

. Changes in hygiene or look

. Increased isolation in social conditions

. Way of speaking or writing this is abnormal or nonsensical

. A trade in persona. Irrational, bitter, or worried responses to loved ones.

. Inability to sleep or listen.

. Inappropriate or uncommon behavior

. Extreme state of affairs approximately religion and the occult.

Positive symptoms and signs

Disturbances which might be brought to the person of the individual.

. Illusions - misconceptions - humans might also additionally accept as true with that a person is spying on them, or that they're someone famous

. Hallucinations- Seeing, feeling, tasting, being attentive to or smelling something that virtually does now not exist. The most common experience is paying attention to imaginary voices giving instructions or making comments to the person.

. Disrupted speech and thinking - shifting from difficulty rely to trouble count, meaninglessly. They make up their non-public terms and sounds.

Negative signs

Negative signs and symptoms are capabilities which can be "loss" of the individual's personality.

. Alienation

. Extreme apathy.

. Lack of motivation or initiative

. Lack of Emotional Responses

Chapter 13: The Five Kinds Of Schizophrenia

1. Paranoid Schizophrenia

The character feels distinctly suspicious, persecuted, or has feelings of grandiosity, or feels a mixture of these feelings.

2. Disorganized Schizophrenia

The individual is frequently incoherent in speech and thinking, but can also don't have any illusions.

three. Catatonic schizophrenia

The person is alienated, silent, terrible and regularly assumes very bizarre body positions.

4. Residual schizophrenia

The man or woman not reviews illusions or hallucinations, but does not revel in motivation or interest in existence.

5. Schizoaffective illness

The character has every symptoms of schizophrenia and of a exquisite temper disease which includes despair.

Chapter 14: Types Of Social Useful Resource Inside The Network For Human Beings And Own Family Members With Schizophrenia

Social assist for the character with schizophrenia

It is important on the way to recognize that you can't do all of it on my own and without help. You are going to want someone that will help you with such things as taking your loved one on a date, bringing him food, going to the films, or buying. It is vital that you put together a help plan for the person with schizophrenia.

. Respite care (ask your health practitioner or social worker)

. A list of friends and own family who've provided their help.

. Employ a care coordinator (an instance, paid a coordinator 100 greenbacks for 5 hours to create a care plan for the only which you love

. Other styles of assist (shelter employees).

Social manual for the caregiver

It can be bodily and mentally laborious traumatic for a person with schizophrenia The extra help you've got were given, the better your capacity to offer exceptional care

Some mind of in which to trying to find help

Join a assist company of different caregivers

Contact the National Alliance for Mental Illness for programs to assist the caregiver of people with intellectual contamination

Contact the Schizophrenia Anonymous Hotline

Talk to circle of relatives contributors, therapists and church personnel in case you sense beaten, or distinctly exhausted.

Self Care

. Exercise 30 minutes an afternoon each day
...

. Eat healthful, balanced meals ...

. Practice relaxation strategies.

. Spend time collectively along with your pals.

. Get enough sleep.

. Get involved in social sports.

. Practice intellectual and breathing strategies.

. Keep a high-quality humorousness.

. Do not use alcohol or tablets.

Chapter 15: The Crisis Plan

Do you have got got a catastrophe plan? Monitor for early signs and symptoms and signs and symptoms of relapse, These are: insomnia, social isolation, lousy personal hygiene, paranoia, hostility and hallucinations.

Every caregiver of a person with schizophrenia need to have a plan in case of a disaster. For instance:

. A listing of all contacts - have the numbers of the health practitioner, psychiatrist, counselor, and family and friends available to provide childcare if wished.

. A plan for a manner to deal with an acute catastrophe - stay calm, validate the reason of his psychosis (fear). Do no longer argue about his delusions and steer the verbal exchange to a safer task count number.

. A plan to get him assist- Suggest travelling the scientific medical doctor for a particular symptom inclusive of insomnia; If he resists, permit him choose out which professional he wants to see just so he feels extra on top of things.

. Discuss the disaster plan on the identical time as the man or woman is not having a crisis. This will help him enjoy much less threatened at the equal time as he's already inside the situation.

. Keep a symptom pocket e-book so you can inform whilst subjects have changed and the relapse has commenced.

Chapter 16: Housing Lodging For People With Schizophrenia

A individual with schizophrenia dreams a sturdy vicinity to stay. Deciding in that allows you to rely on how nicely they might address themselves and what form of supervision they require.

Living with the caregiver is nearly normally the first-rate feasible alternative, so long as the character does not have intense troubles that require a greater supervised environment, which includes substance abuse, refusing to take their medicinal drugs, or every other behavior trouble. If you stay with one in all a type humans, it's miles important to take into account the effect on them, particularly on children.

Another preference includes a residential treatment remedy or a 24-hour facility, a hard and fast domestic, or a building with supervised apartments.

Keep in mind that your feature as a caregiver is drastically crucial to the man or woman with schizophrenia. In a literal feel, you may be the satisfactory character helping him keep a process and a safe haven, which might be some of the horrific results of his infection (jobless/homeless).

You must take delight within the artwork you are doing and recognize how vital and crucial it's miles. Never underestimate the distinction you are making in that character. The effect you have got got made in his life due to your assist and useful resource.

Chapter 17: Types Of Mental Illness.

Agoraphobia- Irrational worry of open spaces, which includes massive avenues, parks or natural environments.

Bipolar - exaggerated changes in temper from mania to most critical despair. Emotional instability.

Anorexia Nervosa- An obsession with controlling the quantity of food you eat.

Bulimia Nervosa- After consuming a big quantity of meals, the individual attempts to get rid of the ingested food from their body thru purgative behaviors (vomiting).

Narcissistic Personality- The man or woman has an inordinate experience of self-significance, a deep need for excessive attention and admiration, relationships, and a loss of empathy for others. However, within the again of that mask of excessive safety, there can be a touchy vanity this is prone to the slightest complaint.

Paranoia- It is a disease characterised through one or more delusions. That is to mention, that those humans are honestly satisfied of factors that are not real. For example, someone is chasing them to harm them.

Depression

It is a highbrow sickness characterized via a country of chronic disappointment, lack of hobby in taking component in sports activities affecting their each day lifestyles.

Anxiety

It is a highbrow ailment characterized with the useful resource of a regular fear of hysteria or worry so sturdy and continual that it interferes along with your each day lifestyles.

Bipolar

It is a sickness characterised through modifications in mood starting from depression to exaggerated pleasure.

Compulsive obsession

Obsessive mind that reason repetition of (compulsive) behaviors.

Post-annoying syndrome

A sickness wherein the individual has issue recovering after experiencing or witnessing a traumatic event.

Attention-deficit / hyperactivity disease

A chronic situation that consists of trouble focusing, hyperactivity, and impulsivity.

The maximum commonplace highbrow disorders are:

. Anxiety issues - panic, compulsive obsession.

. Depression- Bipolar- and others of the country of mind.

. Eating issues

. Personality troubles.

. Post-traumatic pressure infection

. Psychotic troubles- schizophrenia

Vocabulary / phrase list

Tardive dyskinesia

It is a worried machine infection that reasons repetitive actions, specifically of the mouth, which incorporates mouth twisting and lip smacking, that a person can not manipulate. It is sort of constantly due to long-term use of the older types of psychoactive medicinal pills used to cope with a few highbrow health conditions, collectively with schizophrenia and bipolar disorder. Tardive dyskinesia additionally can be due to metoclopramide.

Chapter 18: Schizophrenia And Mortality

People with schizophrenia die at an in advance age than exclusive healthy people. Men with this illness are 5.1% more likely to die than the rest of the population, and women five.6%.

Suicide is the most commonplace contributor to this determine as suicide is 10% to 13% better in human beings with schizophrenia.

The severe melancholy and psychosis they undergo because of not being treated. Other people are:

.Accidents- Although just a few of the humans with this example power a car, research show that they've two times the threat of having a automobile twist of destiny or being hit by means of using using a automobile.

. Diseases- Evidence indicates that they be bothered through greater infections, coronary coronary heart illness, diabetes II, and breast maximum cancers (in ladies) than the rest of the population. People with schizophrenia who grow to be sick are lots a good deal less capable of describe their signs and symptoms and signs and symptoms to their medical doctors, and a number of the medical doctors take delivery of as authentic with that the signs and symptoms and symptoms are a part of their intellectual contamination. There is also proof that human beings with schizophrenia have a excessive tolerance for ache and have a tendency no longer to are trying to find scientific help until the illness has superior sufficient to be handled.

. Homeless- Apparently there may be an illustration that homeless people have a immoderate loss of life fee due to the fact this causes them to be greater at risk of contamination and accidents.

Schizophrenia is a chronic brain disease that affects plenty a great deal much less than 1% of america population. When the sickness is lively, the signs and signs and signs and symptoms may additionally moreover moreover consist of delusions, hallucinations, disorganized speech (nonsensical), difficulty questioning and lack of motivation. But with the proper treatment and medicines the signs and signs can beautify appreciably and the opportunity of each other catastrophe decreases..

Even regardless of the fact that there may be no treatment for this ailment, the experts are coming across the reasons of this disorder with the study of genetics, the usage of images of the mind and present process behavioral studies.

Chapter 19: What Is Schizophrenia?

My personal definition of schizophrenia is that it's miles a very excessive and persistent intellectual contamination that proper now impacts the victim by using the usage of using inflicting them to "loss contact with fact". According to the Mayo Clinic, schizophrenia is "a disorder that affects someone's ability to think, sense, and behave surely".

We have all heard the phrases such as "break up thoughts" and "cut up person". But those are deceptive labels, together with others we have got all heard, "loopy, basket-case, looney, insane". Often, society places labels on what they do not understand, and that is how myths develops. Myths are then spread through gossip due to worry or spite. This then becomes the worldwide stigma that exists nowadays. The excellent way to stop this stigma is through recognition, beginning with education.

We all realise that this ailment has existed all the time, but it wasn't defined, till 1887, as a awesome highbrow infection with the aid of a medical doctor named Emile Kraepelin. Before that point, all and sundry termed as "bizarre" come to be positioned into one single class. This category blanketed all the mentally unwell and developmentally disabled. Obviously, there was not as an entire lot studies finished at that factor as there may be now. And I consider there is a lot more absolutely everyone need to understand about highbrow contamination, in particular schizophrenia. With time, increasingly more studies can be finished and there may be a much better information of the signs and symptoms, remedies, and of the sickness itself.

Throughout time, all "weird" humans had been placed in "insane asylums" for a "lifestyles-term". By 1955, 4 out of every 1000 people had been in highbrow hospitals. Gradually, deinstitutionalization became enacted and slowly patients were reintroduced into society. Group homes then have become extra severa.

Electroconvulsive Shock Therapy changed into used, inside the beyond, as a manner to "control" sufferers who have been no longer experiencing fantastic behavior adjustments with medicine. At that point, there have been moreover lobotomies performed, in which part of the affected individual's thoughts have become removed. ECT isn't always regularly though used these days, and within the United States lobotomies are certainly nearly non-existent.

The essential treatment for schizophrenia is antipsychotic remedy. The first treatment turned into designed for schizophrenics in 1952, through Dr. Henri Laborit. It became referred to as chlorpromazine, moreover known as Thorazine. It changed into authorized with the resource of the Food and Drug Administration in 1954. Doctors noticed excessive first rate modifications in the schizophrenic patients' behaviors, and it additionally delivered on a reduction of the signs and symptoms that the troubled incurred.

So, you possibly be thinking what the signs of schizophrenia are. This might be discussed in the subsequent economic spoil.

Chapter 20: Symptoms Of Schizophrenia

People with schizophrenia enjoy a big sort of signs and symptoms concerning disruptive and bizarre mind, behaviors, moods, speech, and mental outcomes.

The signs and symptoms maximum human beings partner with schizophrenia are:

Delusions. Delusions are false beliefs that the victim interprets to be actual and right. The 3 critical topics that the ones delusions revolve round are authorities, intercourse, and religion. But a victim should have delusions about something in any respect. I do agree with that the ones delusions stem from the subconscious mind, based totally definitely mostly on some beyond enjoy that the sufferer located unsettling to his or her thoughts. Paranoia (questioning a person is out to get you or is speaking at the back of your lower decrease lower back) is clearly just a form of a myth. I need to stress proper proper right here that a person experiencing delusions in reality believes them to be actual, due to the fact their mind will use some thing it could to rationalize their fake beliefs. It is only a top part of this very vital intellectual infection.

Hallucinations. In my own terms, I outline a hallucination as a faux sensation, going on with the sight, scent, contact, taste, or paying attention to schools of the victim. Most generally, hallucinations arise with the listening to. A schizophrenic individual can pay interest voices that aren't definitely there. But in their mind, the voices are real, and they hold to believe this no matter their friends, households, and clinical doctors trying to provide an explanation for that those voices don't exist to truly every body however the sufferer herself. The second maximum commonplace hallucination impacts the texture of sight. A character will see subjects that in reality are not there, which encompass an inanimate item, a few problem transferring, or likely some thing "reworking" into some element else.

Hallucinations of contact, smell, and taste are uncommon, but they do get up in intense times.

Disorganized thoughts and speech. Schizophrenics are not able to pay interest on a topic and often ramble on from concern recall to situation be counted and could carry up something this is absolutely beside the factor to the existing conversation. They are not capable of maintain on the proper song as to what is taking place round them. I agree with that that is due to the sufferer's consciousness at the voices in their head. A character thinks the voices are extra important to take note of then to what's taking place within the "actual worldwide." In fact, to a victim the arena that their schizophrenia created for them, is extra real than the "real worldwide".

Abnormal frame moves. A sufferer can also reduce themselves to the level of a toddler. They also can have no motor coordination and may showcase random actions that are not based totally completely in fact. Also, their behaviors appear to have no basis in truth, and they may appear to occur in a random nature.

Inability to complete everyday every day activities. Due to the quantity of highbrow struggling this is taking vicinity in the mind of a schizophrenic affected person, they may be now not able to paintings. They can be not able to attend to their non-public non-public desires, which incorporates showering or perhaps eating. They may be extremely socially and emotionally awkward. It may additionally furthermore even be so immoderate that they'll be not able to revel in some thing in any respect in lifestyles.

A symptom I want to strain, that isn't always addressed often enough in scientific books, is the extreme worry that a schizophrenic person may moreover furthermore experience. Imagine being inside the shoes of someone who fears for their lifestyles on a chronic basis. Their mind may additionally additionally have concocted the idea that everyone is out to kill them. These delusions are most effective extra desirable via the victim's hallucinations which will be predisposed to verify the validity of the faux beliefs.

People who be concerned with the resource of schizophrenia definitely do have a completely impaired reputation of even having the contamination. How can they healing the difficulty that is affecting their mind, after they want a healthful mind to restore it? It's a lure 22. At least if you have an contamination that isn't "intellectual" in class, you may use your mind to are searching out the perfect treatment for that contamination.

Chapter 21: Causes Of Schizophrenia

Why do humans get this awful and disheartening highbrow contamination? Is it their very very very own fault? Do you deserve it? Why is that this happening to me?

I would really like to strain that this isn't always your fault in any manner by any method. You did not some thing to deserve this. You are not "vulnerable-minded" or "inadequate". Schizophrenia is sincerely only a bodily contamination that occurs to have an effect on the brain.

Schizophrenia can be due to plenty of problems. Most usually it is perception to get up because of "terrible biology" concerning the mind. Using a number of mind scans and imaging strategies, scientists and docs have observed versions within the thoughts shape, which encompass a discounted amount of gray consider and an normal period of the amygdala, of their sufferers who've schizophrenia.

Schizophrenia may be due to chemical defects in the mind. The neurotransmitters, "wiring on your thoughts" that transmits messages, may not be functioning effectively.

Genetics also can play a issue. It can also run in families, in all likelihood a faulty gene. So basically, if one or both of your parents have schizophrenia, you're extra vulnerable to suffering from it as properly.

Prenatal issues are also idea to cause a person getting schizophrenia within the destiny. Possibly the little one did no longer get enough oxygen, or the mom used tablets throughout the gestation duration.

Use of medication with the useful resource of the schizophrenic themselves may also additionally have moreover been a issue in them getting this mental contamination.

Schizophrenia may be the forestall stop result of early surroundings. Possibly a tough past or a demanding revel in also can effect the risk of getting the infection or might also moreover intensify the signs and symptoms that the infection motives.

Past or gift abuse is thought to be a purpose as nicely.

A individual's "social help network", or lack of, may additionally furthermore contribute to this contamination.

Other elements may additionally moreover embody strain and insufficient vitamins.

As studies maintains, so will our statistics of this ailment. And probably one day, medical medical doctors and scientists may be extra capable of pinpoint why the sickness takes place. I genuinely wish they're capable of achieve a higher understanding of the contamination and of its motives. This will cause higher remedy, consisting of latest varieties of treatment and higher remedy for human beings with schizophrenia. Possibly and with any luck, they'll find out a manner to save you this sickness altogether!

Chapter 22: My Battle With Schizophrenia

Schizophrenia need to have introduced at the loss of life of me. I went thru the searing flames of Hell, and I almost died generally due to this thinking about intellectual illness. There had been truly a few years in which I notion I will be killed, both by using others or through manner of my very very personal hand. . . But I decided what I wanted to show it round. I beat all the given odds and now I actually have a danger to live all over again.

I advanced this infection in my early 20s. I be given as right with that the excessive stress that I changed into setting myself beneath contributed to the disorder showing its unsightly face. I changed into pushing myself too difficult in every element of my life. I wasn't getting the right sleep. I concept I need to accomplish a few aspect and the entirety, probable due to mania and my immoderate preference to preserve the sector.

My first sign of the schizophrenia felt like a bomb going off in my head, like a completely sharp pain in a particular location in my mind. Then the delusions, hallucinations, and paranoia observed.

I began questioning that people have been speaking approximately me due to the reality I can also want to honestly concentrate what they have been saying. I even have emerge as taking note of "voices" and I assumed they have been based totally completely in fact. In reality, they have been very real to me because of the truth that's what my feel of being attentive to have turn out to be telling me.

The voices handiest superior my paranoia. I began to simply receive as right with that human beings had been going to kill me due to the fact I become homosexual. The voices were screaming at me threating rape and homicide. I assumed the voices have been telling me the reality. I lived in fear for my very existence for 11 years. It's not smooth living with the priority u may be assaulted and killed, and for 11 years! Wow, I don't even recognise how all and sundry can do that, however I did!

I went inner and out of psychiatric hospitals and treatment facilities for years. The docs and nurses stored asking me if I become taking note of voices. I normally answered with a "no", due to the reality I endured to keep in mind that the voices have been actual. I idea to myself that I changed into now not loopy, and those need to be real voices speakme to me via a radio transmitter in my lower once more. I idea it modified into a few new era that the authorities turned into the use of to torture people.

With time the delusions have end up increasingly fact based definitely absolutely, as I turned into looking for every manner viable to certainly take shipping of that those "false ideals" have been real. I had delusions about almost the whole thing, and my paranoia have grow to be hovering. I end up experiencing hallucinations of all 4 of my special senses as well. And the hallucinations simplest strengthened the validity of my delusions.

I have end up a huge wide variety. My mind became without a doubt out of manage. I changed into doing crazy topics, due to the truth I feared for my life and I changed into on a quest to reveal to the area that the authorities changed into in reality seeking to kill me via electric powered powered shocks. I believed the perps had been taking pics these electric powered waves at me through the partitions on my apartment so one can stop me from being gay. They had been mission a take a look at to look if they could flip me without delay.

So, this chaotic and agonizing life persevered. No one may also want to understand what have become taking vicinity to me, not even me. I become residing in Hell. There became nowhere to run because of the reality the perps typically located me and have been constantly screaming, threatening, and harassing me with their voices and shock remedy. It simply felt like someone have come to be unexpected me. I felt it usually in my head but precise places in my frame as properly.

Anyways, this insanity went on for many years. I had no idea what modified into actual and what have end up not. I attempted desperately to validate my thoughts, however my delusional horror story ought to no longer allow me to overcome it. My psychosis modified into at a completely lethal diploma.

Then came that fateful day. I grow to be actually out of my mind. And then it took place. . . The next trouble I knew I changed into hospitalized, jailed, and then re-hospitalized in a country forensics middle.

After months of treatment, I changed into capable of get maintain of my contamination and artwork on my coping abilties. I preferred desperately to get higher and be resilient. So, I knew I needed to artwork hard on myself, in order that I have to acquire mental balance yet again.

I fought my conflict to the tremendous of my ability, and I did make it thru. There had been commonly once I concept I even have grow to be a goner. But I modified into capable of discover the braveness, energy, faith, and want to overcome this, which have become the toughest warfare that I ever needed to combat. I "soldiered" on. I am most in fact a warrior. I became the handiest who in no way gave up!

Chapter 23: How To Conquer Your Schizophrenia

Believe it or now not, you can beat this terrible contamination. Please don't forget about that. It will take artwork. Yes, pretty some tough and painstaking paintings. But you can do it! I need to percentage the skills I even have implemented in my private struggle with schizophrenia. These are the abilities that enabled me to emerge from my madness.

Admit there can be a problem. This isn't easy for a variety of people to do. We may also additionally experience inadequate via admitting we've got a mental trouble, because of the stigma linked to it with the useful resource of way of society. But now may be the time to fear about your self and frankly who cares what others say. Those who accept as actual with the stigma are ignorant and genuinely because it is not our fault that we've got schizophrenia, it is not their fault that they stay in lack of awareness. So, if you assume you could have a problem, don't be ashamed to admit it to your self and others.

Accept your contamination. Once you make a decision that a problem exists, you want to considerably take delivery of that interior your coronary heart, soul, and mind. It is what it's far. And as soon as you take shipping of it, you can glide ahead to the subsequent step of handling it.

Get enough relaxation. Sleep is critical for everyone, however even greater so for folks who be through this infection. Set up a ordinary sleep cycle. Avoid naps. Take a damage each time you want to. We all deserve proper rest. It recharges our inner battery.